This book is dedicated to all cyclists who ride their bikes for transport as well as for pleasure, and to the increasing number who will do so in the future.

Together you will help to make the world a better place.

Thank you.

Contents

Introduction

The experience of COVID-19, the precautions taken to avoid catching, transferring and therefore spreading the disease, changed the way we live, and aspects of that change are here to stay. The experience made us reflect on how we live and move, how we look after ourselves and others, and something COVID-19 brought into harsh focus: how we maintain our health and well-being, both individually and collectively. Things will be different in the future and cycling has a big role to play, especially for those who live, commute and move around in our towns and cities.

Cycling also has a crucial part to play in the health of our planet. Global warming is an even bigger threat than COVID-19 and possible future viruses, but one less tangible, so it seems less imminent. Most scientists who have studied global warming and its effects on our environment agree that we need to change the way we live, create less waste and cut emissions that are still a consequence of the way we sustain ourselves. The way we work, eat, travel and what we consume have to change to reduce emissions and secure our future, and that of generations to come. The change has to happen, and the COVID-19 experience will accelerate that change.

During lockdown we saw what the world was like with reduced emissions. We saw clearer skies, the birds sang louder, we even smelled and tasted things as they are, not as they taste and smell when tainted by chemicals in our air that shouldn't be there. The pace of life was slower too, but many of those who could work found they were no less efficient. Working from home opened more eyes to virtual meeting platforms, reducing the number of journeys we take. And those who had to travel found it quicker and more efficient on roads with fewer motor vehicles, especially cars, a very inefficient form of personal transport. Mass transport was once seen as a solution to roads clogged with motor vehicles, and to reducing emissions, but COVID-19 also changed that, which is where the bicycle comes in.

There is no doubt that in its early stages, mass transport and the way we live, work and shop helped spread the virus. We cannot continue travelling every day in the way we did as it leaves us so vulnerable; cycling can help us go forward and build a safer, healthier, less damaging environment. It can even help create a gentler, kinder world. Cycling can improve our physical and mental health, something many knew already, but others discovered during the period of social distancing, when cycling provided much needed exercise. It also puts us in touch with our inner child; cycling was something most found joy in as kids, and enjoying some things with a child's wonder is never a bad thing.

The UK government along with others around the world has recognised the growing importance of cycling, and is working on initiatives of its own, and with other groups and bodies, to make our roads and urban infrastructure more cycle-friendly than ever. In the background, more ambitious plans for active transport, that's walking and cycling, will be rolled out and put in place. This will encourage more people to cycle to work and back, and make cycling part of their and hopefully their families' lives.

Governments know that cycling is a key part of the efforts to restart our economies, because not only is cycling a very efficient way to travel short distances, it's easy to do so while maintaining social distancing, a necessity in preventing COVID-19 or a similar virus spreading out of control again. Governments want people to cycle to work and back, cycle to school, and families to cycle like never before, and most are determined to help facilitate that.

Cycling has a great future and will be part of many more lives than it is now, even though things aren't all they could be for cycling in urban areas in the UK and many other places around the world at the moment. This is being addressed: some perfect urban environments for cycling exist, and many more will come. We are in the early part of a transition from streets and urban infrastructure designed around motor transport, especially the car, to prioritising active transport.

People want to get to and from work by bike, they want to cycle to the shops, do errands and ride to school and back, as well as fit cycling into longer journeys by riding from their homes to a rail station, then cycling to their destination at the other end of their journey. Work has begun to help them. Cycling has a part to play in making our urban areas safer, quieter and healthier; it's good for our personal health and wellbeing, too.

Still, urban infrastructure built around active transport, walking and cycling, is in the future. *Safe Cycling in the City* addresses things as they are now. It's not a book about a cycling nirvana: it provides guidance and advice to help cyclists stay safe on urban streets and cycle-ways now. In some towns and cities, conditions for cycling are great, while others are in a period of transition with an increasing number of pop-up cycle lanes and other spaces that favour cycling. This trend will spread rapidly, but cyclists still encounter other road users, and this book is written with the current road situation in mind.

Safe Cycling in the City will give you the confidence, skills and information you need to cycle on urban roads and cycle-ways. It contains in-depth advice on buying a bike and setting it up to suit you and your needs. That's how people new to cycling should start out, because a bike that suits the purpose to which you put it, a bike that fits you and is set up for you, is a bike that gets ridden. The book then explains how to care for your bike, check it and get the most from it. It will also take you through some simple cycle-maintenance steps to cure common problems, make adjustments and ensure your bike will run smoothly and not let you down.

I review the current situation by briefly explaining why cycling is a transport and health solution. The book then presents the environmental and economic benefits of cycling. It will help you to buy the right bike for you, set it up properly and care for it. *Safe Cycling in the City* also explains the many accessories available to cyclists, what you need and how to buy it, as well as providing a guide to the best clothing to wear in different climates.

The right bike, equipment and clothing will help you not just cope with urban cycling, but enjoy it. Just as important is learning the skills that will help you ride safely and confidently. Confidence is a crucial factor in safe urban cycling, and so is successfully integrating with other road users. The skills you will learn or be refreshed on in this part of the book are crucial for your safety, and will greatly increase your enjoyment of cycling in urban areas. I also provide tips on cycling in various weather conditions.

I show you how to choose a route, and how to find out about help and resources for cyclists and cycling. Finally, I look at health and fitness, how cycling helps improve both, and the book ends with a look at how to deal with any problems, physically or with your bike, that you may encounter.

Safe Cycling in the City is a book about using bicycles to travel to work and school, to go shopping and make visits, and to run errands. Cycling can make our lives safer, more enjoyable and much healthier, both physically and mentally, while reducing human impact on the planet. This is above all a practical book, but it's a hopeful, maybe inspirational, one too. It is the twenty-first-century urban and commuting cyclist's handbook.

Chapter 1

....

Why cycle?

....

Cycling has so much to offer. You can explore on a bike, it's a fitness machine, a sport, but perhaps most importantly for everybody living now and for future generations, you can do everyday journeys by bike that you would normally do on public transport or in a private car. That saves you time and money, helps the environment, and you get fit and boost your health all at the same time. Cycling is so good in so many ways that a better title for this chapter might be 'Why not cycle?'.

A bicycle carries you, so its range is far greater than the two other main forms of active transport, walking and running. Cycling is gentle on the joints. You can take it up at almost any age. And it's a great way to get around our towns and cities, in which the average journey is quite short.

During the time we now call 'lockdown', lots of people got on their bikes to do journeys that they would normally have done on public transport or in cars. At a coronavirus briefing on 4 June 2020, the UK Transport Secretary Grant Shapps, talking about a 'green transport revolution', said: 'Despite fewer people travelling overall during this crisis, we've seen around a 100 per cent increase in weekday cycling, and at weekends the increase has been up to around 200 per cent compared to pre-COVID-19 levels.'

The reduction in vehicle traffic was a window on a possible future, a future where people use bikes for work and recreation. That future is where the Earth needs to be for all our sakes. And cycling is fun – many knew that already but many more discovered it during lockdown. The increase in weekday bicycle use was perhaps to be expected, although it was still large, but the weekend increase meant that whole families were cycling, using bikes to explore where they live. By the looks on the faces of the many I saw, they were enjoying it too.

At the launch of the charity UK Cycling's annual Bike Week in June 2020, the Minister of State for Transport, Chris Heaton-Harris, said: 'COVID-19 has made us rethink how we work, shop and travel, and we have seen so many people over the past couple of months discovering or rediscovering a love of cycling as they look for new ways to get around.'

Cycling is an environmentally friendly form of transport with major health benefits, it improves the quality of the air that we breathe, and it helps people get fit and stay healthy, but it does so in a benign way that removes a lot of the 'no pain no gain' ethos connected to many forms of exercise. Cycling is fun, it was something we did as kids. If we can get fit and improve the quality of life for everyone living and working in urban areas while having fun, what's not to like about cycling?

The fact that cycling is good for you has been made official in the light of the COVID-19 pandemic. The advice of both the UK government and the World Health Organization is to cycle or walk when you can, rather than use public transport. Being outdoors rather than in enclosed spaces with others means you are less likely to be exposed to the COVID-19 virus, or risk spreading it to others. The same goes for other infectious diseases.

It's early days yet but the UK government and many local authorities see cycling as the solution to congested and polluted urban areas, and are making changes to our towns and cities so that they are more cycle-friendly. Many people are put off cycling in busy, built-up areas because they fear other road users. Long term that fear will be removed by segregating motor and active transport, with more and more cycle lanes and cycle-only rights of way. But this book is written for now, and the advice in it will help you enjoy cycling and feel safer and more confident on our town and city streets as they are now.

Cycling is a great way to lose weight. It's a low-impact, adaptable exercise that can burn 400 to 750 calories an hour, depending on your weight, speed and the type of cycling you're doing. And what other exercise mode can be used to commute to work or school and back, visit people and places, and run errands? Yes, you can run places, and it's good for you too, but you can travel much further on two wheels than two feet, and with less effort. That makes cycling a practical form of transport as well as exercise.

One of the most common reasons you hear for not exercising is, 'I haven't got time.' If you can't fit the gym around your busy work, home and social life then a fifteen-minute each-way cycle to work and back would meet the government's recommended guidelines for exercise of 150 minutes a week. You also save a fortune in gym membership fees.

Cycling saves you money in other ways too. There's a bike to buy if you don't have one, of course, but buying secondhand is good (more about that in Chapter 3), and if you want to buy one there is help through Cyclescheme, an employee benefit scheme that saves you between 25 and 39 per cent on the cost of a bike and accessories. You pay nothing up front and payments are taken tax efficiently from your salary by your employer (see www.cyclescheme.co.uk for details). Bike2Work is another scheme where you can get financial help with the initial costs of cycling (see www.bike2workscheme.co.uk for details).

After the initial outlay you have some running costs, but they are minimal. Tyres wear out, as do other components, but not at any great rate. All told, the cost of buying and running a perfectly serviceable bike for urban journeys is a drop in the ocean compared to running a car, which is at its least efficient on short journeys. A cyclist can ride for well over 2,000 miles on the calorie equivalent of a gallon of petrol.

Not only that, but in urban areas cycling is often quicker than taking public transport or driving. In surveys and tests the world over, cycling regularly comes out as the quickest mode of transport in towns and cities. And because cyclists take only a fraction of the space motorists do, more cyclists on our streets means less road space taken per person so we all get around quicker.

Cycling is a very effective way of increasing your health and wellbeing. Cycling as little as 20 miles a week can reduce your risk of coronary heart disease by half. That's 20 miles in total, so ten 2-mile commutes will do it. That's 4 miles, five days a week. Do more and you reap even more health benefits. And you will do more: cycling is like that, it hooks you, it's a bug you will want to catch.

A 2017 study by the University of Glasgow found that people who regularly cycle to work have a 41 per cent lower risk of dying from all causes. Another study of more than 260,000 people found that those who cycled to work had a 45 per cent lower risk of developing cancer, compared to those who commuted by car or public transport.

Cycling can also help to increase your productivity, which keeps the people you work for happy and benefits the economy. A study found that, on average, people who cycle to work take one less sick day per year than their non-cycling colleagues, saving the UK economy almost £83 million. As well as making you fitter, being outside in the sunshine on your way to work boosts your vitamin D levels, which benefits your immune system, brain and bones.

You see news items all the time about a growing obesity problem, about big increases in Type 2 diabetes sufferers. Cycling can ward off that and many other diseases, helping make Britain a fitter nation. It's often hard for people who are overweight to start exercising, but cycling is perfect exercise for anyone who might have put on a few pounds. The bike carries a person's bodyweight, the rider just pushes the pedals, so there's little risk of the joint problems associated with jogging, for example.

Cycling also has a positive effect on mental health. A Cycling UK survey of more than 11,000 people found that 91 per cent of participants rated off-road cycling as fairly or very important for their mental health. OK, your route to work will most likely be on roads or cycle-only streets, but it's likely to help you clear your mind and there's still the simple buzz you get when exercising. Try to include riding through a park on your commute to add a little bit of the wild feeling those off-roaders get. Green spaces are good for us.

The 'buzz' is caused by natural substances our bodies produce when we exercise. They are called endorphins and they trigger a positive feeling in the body, similar to the effect of morphine. That's why exercise can be accompanied by a positive and energising outlook on life. Get some of that on the way to work and it sets you up for the day.

Endorphins also act as analgesics, diminishing the perception of pain, and as sedatives so they calm you down. They are manufactured in the brain, spinal cord and other parts of the body, and are released in response to brain chemicals called neurotransmitters. The neuron receptors to which endorphins bind are the same ones that bind some pain medicines. Unlike with morphine, however, the activation of these receptors by the body's endorphins does not lead to addiction or dependence. Regular exercise reduces stress, wards off anxiety and feelings of depression, boosts self-esteem and can even improve the quality of sleep you get.

We are developing a 24/7 state of heightened awareness, and certainly many of us spend long hours looking at screens. Disconnecting from all that's going on and falling asleep is a struggle for many people. Exercise can help with that. A study by the University of Georgia of more than 8,000 people found a strong correlation between cardio-respiratory fitness and sleep patterns; a lower level of fitness was linked to both an inability to fall asleep and poor sleep quality. So cycling to work could help you sleep better (at home, of course!).

Cycling can make you cleverer. All exercise increases oxygen to your brain and by doing so reduces the risk of disorders that lead to memory loss, such as diabetes and cardiovascular disease. Exercise may also enhance the effects of helpful brain chemicals and protect brain cells.

Cycling is a great way for kids to start learning about machines, and as they get older it helps them learn about the environment and about fitness. Cycling carries with it practical lessons in engineering, ecology, geography and human biology, and young cyclists who want to race tend to eat healthier and are in less danger from overconsumption of alcohol.

You can eat more, and you'll eat healthier. Ride plenty and you can indulge yourself with treats that no diet would include, so long as you don't overdo it. Having said that, although your appetite will grow as you ride more, it will also change. Left to its own devices, a well-exercised body begins to crave things that are good for it. Ride more and you'll eat healthier.

Cycling can even improve your job prospects. Bristol University carried out a study using 200 people and found that those who exercised before work or at lunchtime improved their time and workload management. Exercise also boosted their motivation and their ability to deal with stress. The study reported that workers who exercised felt their interpersonal performance improved, they took fewer breaks and found it easier to finish work on time. Another survey found that slimmer people tend to earn more money. In fact, they said that each single-point drop in body mass index (BMI), albeit a very crude measurement of weight against height, represented £800 more earned per year per person on average.

Bosses know this. They know exercise improves work performance, and cycling is an incredibly effective way of exercising during the working day because you can use a bike to commute to work. More and more businesses are fitting showers, changing rooms with lockers and secure bike-storage areas to facilitate this.

More people cycling and less using motor transport to get around our towns and cities is great news for all of us. Every year in the UK about 40,000 deaths are linked to outdoor pollution, much of it emitted needlessly. In London, it was found that two-thirds of car journeys are less than 3.1 miles (5 km), a distance that can be covered in twenty minutes at a gentle cycling pace. This pattern is seen in many other cities around the UK.

The Olympic gold medallist and world champion Chris Boardman, who is now a leading figure in campaigning for better urban infrastructure for cyclists, has a vision for the communities of the future, which he outlined several years ago. 'I want bikes to be used as transport. I want my kids to be able to ride to school and to the park. I'd like to be able to pedal to the station or to the shops. This can only happen if there are less cars, and people will only use cars less if they are not the easiest solution. So, the key is local governments having a clear and detailed holistic view of what they want their cities to look like in ten years' time,' he said. We are well on the way to achieving that, and progress is accelerating now due to the experience of COVID-19, maybe the only good thing to have come out of that terrible disease.

Replacing short urban journeys in cars or on buses and trains by cycling will help reduce the spread of diseases such as COVID-19, improve our health and fitness, improve our mental health and sense of wellbeing, empower and revitalise us, save us money and improve the environment. Yes, the weather in the UK sometimes isn't the best for cycling, but look at the amount of people who use cycling as transport in other northern European countries, such as Denmark and the Netherlands. It was a wise person who once said that there is no such thing as bad weather, only bad clothes. We'll talk about how to cope with rainy days and what to wear later in the book. So get your bike out, and if you haven't got one the next chapter shows you how to buy the right bike for you.

Chapter 2

Buying a bike

The bicycle is in its third century of development, so you would expect it to be exactly what it is, a sophisticated machine with many variations. At first sight there is a baffling array of bikes on the market, that suit many different uses and environments, but don't let that put you off. Bikes are very adaptable, and although some are designed specifically for riding in urban areas, other types of bikes work very well too, maybe with a few adaptations. The most important thing is to get a bike that fits you, a bike that is robust, and to keep it well maintained. We'll deal with how to buy a bike that fits later in this chapter.

Of course, you might already own a bike, or two, and we'll talk about adapting almost any bike to provide comfortable, safe and easy urban cycling later in the book. For now, let's address the needs of those who haven't got a bike, or just want to buy a bike specifically for urban cycling. Like I said, you've got plenty of choice. For a start, you can buy new or secondhand.

BUYING A NEW BIKE

Bikes designed specifically for cycling in urban environments are the most obvious choice for commuting and urban use. Manufacturers offer a large range of urban or city bikes, both pedal-powered and pedal-powered with supplementary electric power, or e-bikes as they are known. Other bikes good for urban use are hybrid bikes, 'fixies' (the bikes with only one gear ratio preferred by city couriers all over the world because of their lightness and simplicity), and folding bikes, which are perfect if your journey involves other transport modes or if you need to take your bike inside a building with you.

Bikes designed for cycle touring and expeditions are very good too. They are robust and they have fixing points on their frames to which you can attach pannier carriers. Pannier bags are a great way of carrying things on a bike. If you need to carry stuff to and from work, or if your cycle commute is long enough for you to require a change of clothes at work and you need to carry those with you, panniers are a great way of doing that. I'll cover bags and transporting things by bike in full in the next chapter, but if you are going to do that it's always better for the bike to carry the load rather than you, so when you buy your bike it is worth checking it has carrier fixing points.

And to add even more choice there are e-bike versions of hybrid and folding bikes too, both fitted with integral electric motors providing differing levels of power to help you pedal. I'll talk about e-bikes later in this chapter and at various times in the book, but I think I can sum them up now by saying they are very suitable for urban use, and are perfect for anyone not used to cycling.

Road bikes work OK for urban cycling, as do mountain bikes, although both benefit from a change of tyres (more robust tyres in the case of road bikes, and tyres most commonly called 'slicks' instead of the knobbly tread tyres normally found on mountain bikes). Older bikes, often called utility bikes, are good too, although you may have problems buying replacement parts for them.

Road bikes with dropped handlebars really come into their own if you are doing a longer commute. Modern road bikes are light, have a good range of gears and they are perfect if you live outside an urban area and want to commute into a town or city by bike. Because they are light and their tyres have a low rolling resistance, you'll be able to cover longer distances per time unit spent on the bike than most other types of bike. You can even buy sleek-looking road bikes with electric motor assistance.

Mountain bikes are good to ride in urban environments where there are lots of bumpy roads or other rough surfaces to negotiate. You probably only need a front-suspension mountain bike, which cyclists call hardtail bikes, not a full suspension bike. If you buy a hardtail and find you want shock absorption for the rear of the bike, you can get a suspension seat post fitted later.

The frame is the heart of any bike. Bike frames, apart from high-end competition bikes, are made out of welded or brazed metal tubes. The wheels, saddle, handlebars and other equipment fit into or attach to the bike frame. Frames come in different sizes, and it's the frame's size that determines the size of a bike, but more on that later.

You will hear or read the term 'geometry' applied to bike frames. The main thing you need to know about frame geometry is that it refers to the layout of the frame tubes. Each frame tube has a different name, and it's worth knowing them as they will be referred to throughout this book. Here's a simple diagram you can refer to, showing the frame tubes with their names.

A stylised bicycle to show its composite parts

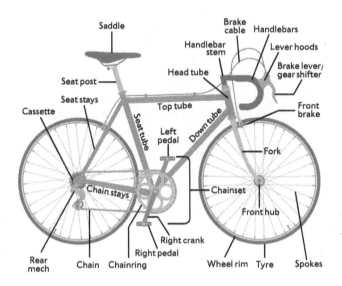

Frame geometry in terms of the proportional length of the various tubes and angles at which they join is a hotly debated subject among enthusiasts, but the main frame geometry consideration for an urban cyclist is whether to go for a bike with a male or female geometry; the latter is also called a 'step-though' frame. Female or step-through frames have the same tubes as the above male example, but the top tube joins the seat tube at a much lower point. Traditionally this low top-tube design was to allow the rider to cycle comfortably while wearing a skirt or dress, but bikes with low top tubes are easier to mount and dismount, which is why they are often called 'step-through' bikes today. Which type of frame you buy is purely a matter of personal choice.

There is another much subtler frame-design variation that women might want to consider when buying a bike, and that is Women Specific Design (WSD). WSD is more commonly associated with road and mountain bikes, and denotes subtle changes in frame-tube proportions and joint angles, and in other equipment on the bike that reflect differences between female and male anatomy. A crucial factor for every woman who cycles, where WSD has to be considered, is in getting the right saddle. I'll deal with WSD saddles in detail in Chapter 4: Are you Sitting Comfortably? For now, no matter what bike you decide to buy, female cyclists should always ensure it either has a WSD saddle fitted, or you have the one already on it swapped for a WSD saddle before you buy the bike. If you are buying secondhand and the bike doesn't have a WSD saddle, you can fit one later.

If you want WSD, you are better buying from a bike shop because they have the knowledge about the subject. It's worth considering seeking good advice in this area, because even among WSD saddles there are design variations. One might suit you a lot better than another, and many shops have female staff who have been trained in WSD and bike fit for women. It's well worth talking to them because the correct saddle makes a world of difference in comfort.

Buying online works fine, although for women there is that saddle question to consider, but you can always visit a shop with your bike later and find the right saddle if the one the bike comes with isn't working for you. If you are buying online I recommend you use retailers who offer the chance to ask questions about the bike you want to buy, either on the phone or through online dialogue.

If you prefer a human touch, however, many bike shops were open throughout the COVID-19 lockdown, so are used to trading in conditions of social distancing and have well thought out in-shop protocols to follow. Bike shops were seen as an essential service by the UK government, which shows how big a splash cycling is on the UK's economic and administrative radar now. And the best bike shops have well-trained staff who are knowledgeable about bike sizing. It pays the shops and the manufacturers to make sure they are, and often both provide training in this area.

Retail is very competitive now, which makes it vital for bike shops to train their staff so they can provide added value with their service. And don't be nervous about asking questions. Even if they are the most obvious questions to an experienced cyclist, the staff of good bike shops understand that if somebody is new to cycling it can all appear very bewildering. But if the staff or the shop make you feel uncomfortable, then that is a window on their service and attitude, so it's probably not a good idea to buy there.

And don't just consider the big chains of bike shops: independent bike shops, family-run businesses many of them, are very good. The ones that survived some of the lean times the bike industry has experienced over the years did so because of their knowledge and excellent customer service. It's even worth paying a bit more for your bike to get their customer care and access the knowledge they have built up over the years. Making friends with your local bike shop is a good idea for any cyclist, and the best way to take advantage of their experience is to buy your bike from one. Customer loyalty is a prize now, and a good business will go out of its way to maintain it.

THE RIGHT SIZE

Bike size is important for many reasons. A bike that is either too small or too big for the person riding it is uncomfortable, but it's also difficult to control; two factors that make it less easy and less safe to ride. You need a bike that is proportional to your height, so your body weight is distributed over the bike optimally. This is a crucial factor in how the bike feels, performs and handles. A bike that feels good and performs and handles well is easy to manoeuvre. You should feel neither stretched nor constricted when riding. The various controls – the brakes, gear shift leaver, e-bike power controls – should all be at your fingertips. As you become more experienced at cycling your bike should feel like an extension of your own body. It's a good feeling, and it means you will be much better balanced, in control and therefore far safer than riding a bike that doesn't fit.

Correct weight distribution means the bike will go where you steer it, and you won't wobble when setting off from a standing start or when removing a hand from the handlebars to make hand signals. With the correct size of bike, you are able quickly and safely to place a foot, or both feet, on the floor whenever you stop. And you have to stop a lot when cycling in some urban areas, for example at road junctions or traffic lights. You will also be able quickly and safely to resume pedalling when you set off, while holding the bike steadily in the right direction, which is really crucial when you are in any traffic. Having a wobbling, unsteady cyclist in front of them often causes drivers to try to get past, even on occasions when that might not be safe. Holding a steady course gives confidence to all around you. It's something you should practise, and I'll go into more detail on how to do all these things in Chapter 6: Cycling skills.

Many aspects of a bike, such as the height and position of the saddle, can and should be adjusted to give the rider a perfect custom fit, and I will talk about those in Chapter 4, but the first and underlying step towards safe, comfortable cycling is to buy the right size bike at the outset. Making adjustments to custom fit your bike is the fine detail of bike fit, the big broad brushstroke is to get the correct size bike for you at the outset.

Bike sizes are determined by the size of their frames, in particular the length of the frame's seat tube. That's the part of the frame that runs from the bottom bracket, which houses the bearings that the pedal cranks revolve around, upwards to the point where the post with the bike's saddle mounted to it fits into the frame. Frame sizes are given as the specific length of the seat tube or as a more general size ranging from extra-extra-small (XXS) to extra-extra-extra-large (XXXL).

Listen to advice on correct sizing supplied by online retailers or in a bike shop. Such advice is mostly supplied by the different bike manufacturers, who know their brand and models best. To give you somewhere to start, however, here is a general guide to what size bike suits a rider of a particular height. The guide is applicable to most urban and e-bikes. Road and mountain bikes have different geometry, although the general size column is a good guide for the size of road or mountain bike that is right for your height.

Bike size guide

Height (feet & inches)	Height (cm)	Mountain Bike Sizes	Road/Urban Bike Sizes	General Sizing
4'8–5'1	143–55	13	44 cm	XXS
5'1–5'4	155–63	15	48 cm	XS
5'4–5'7	163–70	16	51 cm	S
5'7–5'10	170–78	18	54 cm	M
5'10–6'	178–83	19	56 cm	L
6'–6'3	183–91	20	58 cm	XL
6'3–6'5	191–96	21	60 cm	XXL
6'5–6'9	196–205	22	62 cm	XXXL

As I said, the above is for guidance only. It's a place from which to start when buying a new bike, but it will be very useful if you are buying a secondhand bike. Remember, though, bike sizes vary between different designs and manufacturers. Most of them provide a size guide to their bikes, and many manufacturers help train the staff of shops and other outlets that sell their brand. Some manufacturers take other body dimensions, in particular inside-leg length, into consideration when advising on bike size, as do many shops and online retailers. There is a lot of information out there for bike buyers, and it is well worth reading what different manufacturers say about their bikes.

Another good way to check a bike with standard geometry is the right size for you, especially if it's an urban bike, is to stand astride it with both feet flat on the floor and your legs comfortably straight. Don't sit in the saddle, just make sure there is a good gap between the bike's top tube and your crotch. This is an especially useful tip when buying a secondhand bike.

The need to equip yourself with the correct-sized bike can't be overstated. A bike that fits is a not just practical and safe, it's a joy to ride.

BUYING SECONDHAND

At first sight this can be a bit of a minefield, but it doesn't have to be. For a start, there is a growing number of shops in the UK dedicated to selling secondhand bikes, and many others, especially small independent retailers, who sell secondhand bikes as well as new. There are bargains to be had here, because the shops take in old bikes as trade-ins on new bikes, and it pays them to only take bikes in part exchange that are basically sound. They then service the trade-ins and offer them for sale. Buying a bike like that from a reputable bike shop is often a very sound investment. Plus you've made a friend with the shop, which means it's in their interest to look after you so they retain you as a customer.

Some bike shops sell ex-demo and ex-hire bikes, and both can be bargains. The ex-demo bikes have often not been heavily used, while hire bikes might have quite a few miles on them, but they are generally well maintained. Check their tyres, though; if they look worn you might be able to get the shop to swap them for a new pair and include it in the price.

I should talk about tyre wear at this point as it is certainly something you need to consider when buying a secondhand bike. Look around the whole circumference of each tyre, check for excessive wear and cuts in the tread or in the sidewalls, and look for any bulges or deformities in the tyres. They all mean the tyre needs replacing before you start riding, so that should be reflected in the price. There is more about tyres when I look at caring for your bike in Chapter 5.

There is a growing number of bike recycling businesses and charities in the UK that take in old bikes people don't want, then work on them to bring them into sound working order, and either donate them to good causes or sell them. People who work in places such as this are often very committed to what they do, which makes them a good place to buy. In any case, recycling anything is something worth supporting against the background of a rampant consumer society in the Western world. And if you can do that while picking up a genuine bargain, so much the better. Bike recycling centres are a fabulous initiative, well worth searching out on the internet and supporting.

Even if you don't buy from a bike recycling centre, you should offer them any old bikes you no longer use. Some of the charities repair the bikes and send them to places overseas where an old bike may mean a person can travel for education, get work or even set up their own business. It really can be life-changing. There's some fascinating and really worthwhile work being done by bike charities now.

Secondhand online

If you are looking online to buy a secondhand bike there is eBay, which is a good place to look because it has a ratings system for sellers and this can warn you against anybody selling a few bikes secondhand that aren't of very high standard. Also, if you have a problem with the bike or the seller, it's possible to mediate through eBay.

There are many websites dedicated to secondhand bikes and to local cycle sales. There are social media groups where people offer bikes and cycling equipment for sale, too. The key to buying online is to ask lots of questions, and ask to see more photographs if you aren't happy with the ones on show. You need to ask the seller to measure the bike from bottom bracket to the top of the seat tube, too. Then you can consult the bike size guide included earlier in this chapter. That will help you eliminate bikes that are too small or too big for you.

Photos are necessary to find a bike that is worth inspecting in person. Photos help you reject the ones you don't like the look of.

Ask for close-up photos of both sides of the area where the down tube joins the head tube, as well as both sides of where the chain stays join the bottom bracket. Again, the bottom bracket is the lowest part of the frame, where the cranks revolve. It's a good idea to ask for a photo taken from under the bottom bracket too, which is generally where the manufacturer's frame number is located.

No frame number, especially if you can see bare metal where it should be, means it could have been removed because the bike was stolen at some point. Frame numbers are important, and there are several online databases to check them on. The police-approved database is called Bike Register. You could ask the seller for the frame number and check it before you go and see it. If they don't want to do that then it's an alarm bell. Trust your judgement, too: if you don't like the story the seller is telling you, leave it. Buying a stolen bike is not worth the hassle.

Asking for more photos if you are buying online is only the first step to make sure a secondhand bike bought online is worth what you are paying. You have got to see the bike before you buy; photos just help you save making wasted journeys. Once you've decided on a bike you like the look of, go and see it. This is why local sales websites and bike forums are a good place to search for a bike. If you are new to cycling and have a friend who is already cycling and more knowledgeable than you, ask them if they will look at the bike with you. It can save you making a mistake, or they may be able to advise you against buying a bike that's not really suitable for what you want to use it for. An experienced cyclist can also check it's the right size.

Whatever, you must give the bike a close inspection. Lift the front then the rear of the bike, spinning the front wheel first then the rear. If the bike has calliper brakes and the wheel rims catch on the brake pads anywhere around their circumference, then the wheels aren't true and will need correcting. If the catching, referred to in cycling as a 'buckled wheel', isn't too bad it's not a deal breaker, but it will require some work at a bike shop because the buckle reflects an imbalance in the wheel, so it's not safe and will get worse. The cost of any repair should be pointed out to the seller and reflected in the price.

Examine all control cables, that's brake and gear cables, to see if any are frayed. Check the brakes and gears work. Apply the front brake and push the bike forward; if the front wheel still revolves then at the very least the brake needs servicing. Do the same with the rear brake and wheel to see if that needs servicing. Check the handlebars and seat are tight in the frame. Check the tyres for wear, cuts or bulges too.

If you find anything mentioned so far is defective then there will be a cost implication in fixing it, but the bike may still be worth buying, especially if the seller comes down in price. The exception, though, is play in bearings, unless you really know about bikes and judge the defect to be fixable. Any play shows that the bearings are worn, and replacing bearings can be expensive; if the bearing surfaces are worn then the bike isn't worth buying at all. Worn bearings are also a sign that the bike has had a lot of use, without being too closely maintained. It's probably best to avoid a bike with worn bearings, unless you know what you are looking at and can rectify it.

To do a quick bearing check start with the wheels. Grab the front wheel and try to move it at right angles to its normal direction of travel: any movement or looseness in wheel hubs means worn bearings. Revolve the wheel and listen: any clunks from the wheel hub mean the bearings are worn; any squeaks mean their lubrication has gone and they are likely to be worn. Do the same with the rear wheel. Check headset bearings next – they are the bearings that the steering moves on. All you need to do is grab the handlebars, apply the front brake and push the bike forward; any forward movement around the top of the head tube or cracking or creaking sounds mean the bearings are worn. Lastly, check the pedal and crank bearings by grabbing a pedal and applying sideways pressure at right angles to the direction of normal travel. Any sideways play or clunks or creaks mean the bearings are worn and there will be cost implications.

Like all bearing wear, if you know what you are doing and assess the problem as fixable, especially if you get the seller to drop their price, then you might be OK. Anybody else should avoid buying that bike. There are plenty of bargains to be had, so you don't have to buy the first bike you see.

Finally, the big no to buying any bike is if you find defects in the bike's frame. Check it thoroughly. It's crucial you do because to all intents and purposes a problem with the frame means you shouldn't buy the bike. Examine all of the points where the frame tubes join. They are stress points and any cracks you see, even slight ones, render the bike unsafe, so don't buy it. Pay close attention to the chain stays, particularly around the chainset (the large toothed sprocket that is turned by the pedals and in turn drives the bike's chain, and therefore the rear wheel). If there is any damage in that area beyond slight scratches and chips in the paintwork, then don't buy the bike. Don't be afraid to turn the bike upside down, asking the owner's permission of course, to check the underneath of the tubes too. If the owner won't let you then that's another alarm bell. Inspect the whole frame for any cracks or dents, and reject the bike if you see any.

Buying a second-hand mountain bike is slightly more complicated because of their suspension systems. You need to check the way the suspension works, and in the case of full suspension mountain bikes there are many more moving parts you need to look at. If you don't know about mountain bikes and want to buy one, try to take somebody who does know about them with you when you inspect it. Do all the checks recommended above, and include these checks on the suspension.

Check the front suspension by pushing down forcefully on the handlebars with the front brake applied; the suspension should depress and return smoothly without any clunks or clicks. Next, keeping the front brake applied, push forward on the handlebars while looking down on the forks, particularly at the two struts that run down to the wheel hub. Any forward or backward rocking in the suspension indicates a problem inside them, and the forks could be worn out. Look at the bare top part of the suspension struts after you have compressed the forks and allowed them to return; any excess oil on the bare metal parts of the struts, especially if it is dirty oil, means the oil seals aren't working and will need replacing, which in turn is a sign of poor maintenance. All these defects involve extra costs.

Test the rear suspension by pushing down forcefully on the saddle; again the suspension should compress and return smoothly. Look for evidence of leaking oil on the suspension unit too, as visible oil could mean the seals need replacing. Finally, try rocking the suspension by pushing at right angles to the normal direction of travel. There should be no play in pivot points. Play in pivot points means the bearings, or even the pivots themselves, are worn. A bike like that is best avoided.

Paying for secondhand bikes is another thing you need to be careful about and it's worth knowing your rights, which are far fewer than when you buy retail. Where you normally have some protection when buying from a reputable retailer or charity, second-hand sales are very much 'buyer beware'. You buy things 'as seen', another commonly used term in the secondhand market. One solution is to pay with PayPal, which offers some protection. However, there is another pitfall there. Sellers often ask you to designate a PayPal payment as a 'gift' so they don't pay fees to PayPal, but if you do that any protection you had from PayPal goes by the board.

Another warning sign is if the seller asks to meet in a neutral place for you to look at the bike and discuss buying it. It might be that they are doing you a favour and meeting halfway between your two locations, or it could be because they don't want you to know where they live. You will have to use your own judgement, but be aware of a possible reason for them not revealing their address. Ask for it, and see how they react.

OK, at this point you might think I'm trying to put a downer on buying secondhand. I'm not – there are great bargains to be had. I'm just pointing out the things you need to check so you don't get stung. Overall, buying secondhand is a good option, especially if it's from somebody you know quite well. Also, new bike sales are very buoyant at the moment, which means there aren't too many cut-price deals out there, certainly not on new urban bikes. Buying secondhand offers the potential for big savings. Just be careful.

FOLDING BIKES

Folding bikes are ideal for commuters, and for people with little space in which to store a standard bike. A number of different types are available, but all of them can be quickly folded into a package that is easily carried or stored, and can then be reassembled into a serviceable bicycle without the use of tools.

The bikes vary in their sophistication, from basic single-speed models to bikes with multiple gears and integral lighting systems, and carrying capacities. There are even folding mountain, road race and time-trial bikes available. And there are folding e-bikes. All have small wheels, which are essential to the design because wheels cannot be folded. One disadvantage of small wheels is that they give a harsh ride; some bikes overcome this by including a suspension system.

Folding bikes are perfect for commuters who also travel on public transport. There is a growing number of innovative new bikes available in response to the demand from both commuters and people who just want to get away from using their cars.

E-BIKES

E-bikes have a huge role to play in active transport now and in the future. They are the perfect solution for somebody who wants to cycle to work and back, but do so with little more effort than they would make when walking. With pedals and some additional electric power, you can travel much further on an e-bike than you can walk in the same time. That's what makes e-bikes perfect commuter vehicles.

Standard bikes are fine for short commutes in the 1- to 5-mile range. They work well for longer commutes too, if you are used to cycling, or if you take it up and find you really enjoy the challenge. The one drawback, some would say, of pedalling a standard bike on a longer commute, over 5 miles, is that you will probably sweat a bit and therefore need a change of clothes. That's not a problem for some, and thousands of bike commuters either carry a change of clothes with them or have them ready at their destination.

It takes a bit of logistics juggling, which I'll talk about later in the book, but commuting distances of 10 or more miles each way is very doable. I work from home now but I commuted like that for years. But if you don't want to do that, the additional power available from an e-bike means you can avoid having to carry a change of clothes, or have one at your destination, on commutes in the 5- to 10-mile range. E-bikes are perfect for short commutes too. They are a simple and efficient way of getting around urban areas on two wheels quickly and with minimum fuss.

E-bikes combine pedal and electric power – we'll get onto how they do that shortly. First, though, you have to remember to charge an e-bike's battery, so you need to know how many miles the battery on your bike will last. Electric power units on e-bikes are limited by law to an output of 250 watts. Maximum speed while receiving any electric power assistance is limited to 15 miles per hour. Go faster than 15 mph and the motor will stop providing power: it is legs only at that point.

The distance an e-bike can travel under power is determined by the output from the motor's battery over a length of time, which is its watts per hour rating (referred to as WF) or ampere rating (AH). The weather plays a part in battery life in that cold temperatures reduce it, as does the terrain ridden over: hills require more power input so the battery drains quicker. Rider weight is also a factor in battery life between charges. E-bike battery life generally ranges from 27 miles to 70 miles, but a new e-bike will come with full instructions to help you work out the expected battery life of your bike. With that, you can work out how often the battery needs charging and establish a charging routine.

Electric power assistance is provided in two ways depending on where the electric motor is located on the bike. The first location is either on or inside the bike frame. The alternative location is in the rear hub.

Bike-frame motors help to drive the cranks. These motors have inbuilt torque sensors, so they activate only when the rider is pushing down on the pedals. They are very efficient because, with the help of the bike's multiple gears, these motors help cyclists ride up even steep hills without too much effort. They do this by reacting to the amount of pressure the rider exerts on the pedals; more pressure from the rider provokes more power from the motor. In short, the motors sense when the rider needs help. Of the two types of e-bikes, it's the frame motor-powered ones that look the most like standard bicycles. In fact, you can't see any evidence of frame motors on some bikes.

Hub motors propel the rear wheel independently from the rider's pedalling, so they work on demand from the rider; either by operating a pedal-assist control located separately on the bike or by means of a throttle. With many hub-powered e-bikes you can select different levels of pedal assist. The bike's electronics then sense from your pedalling when you need the extra power. Throttles are either thumb or twist-grip operated, and a bike with a throttle doesn't require any pedalling by the cyclist, so you can stop pedalling and coast along totally under electric power if you wish. The speed at which you can coast under electric power only, however, is limited by law. So you won't go very fast in that mode, certainly less than 10 miles per hour, unless you are coasting downhill.

To sum up, the feel of a crank-assist e-bike is more like normal cycling: you just get a bit of help from the motor as and when you need it. Hub-drive e-bikes are more for someone who feels they might need a rest from pedalling now and again. You can buy e-bikes in almost any style of standard bike: urban (standard geometry or low top-tube step-through), road, mountain or folding bike.

Chapter 3

What to wear and other equipment

HELMETS

Helmets aren't compulsory for cyclists so it's a matter of personal choice, but I would recommend wearing a helmet whenever you cycle. OK, a cycling-specific helmet won't cope with a massive impact to your head like, for instance, a motorcycle helmet would. Cycling helmets aren't designed to work in the same way as motorcycle helmets. What cycle helmets do is absorb some of the force of any impact within their structure, so in theory they reduce the force of an impact on your head by the helmet taking the hit and getting damaged.

The theory is that, by absorbing the energy of any knock, cycling helmets reduce the velocity at which your brain, which sits in a sack of fluid inside your skull, impacts with your skull. When the brain impacts the inside of the skull the brain can be bruised, or much worse. It is impacts and the resulting bruises that can cause concussion. The slower the impact, the less bruising. That's the theory.

Some people who have studied cycle helmets don't believe they give the level of protection you might think, and I respect that view. It's probably a good argument for not making wearing a helmet while cycling compulsory. My argument for wearing one, however, is that cycle helmets must give you some protection from a bump on the head. I think the biggest argument for wearing one is that, in my experience, they reduce the effects of a simple tumble in which you might bang your head on the road or another object. And because modern cycle helmets are so light, and I'd argue quite stylish, it's no extra bother to wear one.

Speaking from personal experience of the days when modern lightweight helmets weren't around, I had a simple fall from my bike and suffered a slight head trauma that required a trip to hospital. I wasn't travelling at high speed, nor was I hit by another vehicle. All that happened was my front wheel slipped on a patch of oil in wet weather while I was riding at less than 10 miles per hour. The wheel went from underneath me and I fell off my bike, landed on my shoulder, and the side of my head hit the floor. My gut feeling – and it's only my gut feeling, I've no proof – is that had I been wearing a modern lightweight cycling helmet it would have absorbed some of the impact, but instead my head absorbed it all. I've since had similar falls while wearing a helmet, and not suffered any injury.

Now, while talking about bangs on the head, this might sound like me being fussy and overcautious, but it's not. What follows is an important point. Cycling helmets absorb impact by effectively breaking up the force. So while a biggish bang on the head could result in the helmet being obviously cracked or crushed, a small bump might end with no obvious damage to the helmet. The important point here is that even though there is no sign of damage, the structural integrity of the helmet will have been compromised by the impact. The helmet will no longer be effective at protecting your head, so replace it.

Buying a helmet

First of all, never buy a secondhand helmet. You don't know if it's had a knock, and slight bumps might not show on the surface of the helmet, but they will affect its ability to protect you.

If you are an experienced cyclist and have found a make and model of helmet you really like and trust, then buying online is fine. You know what size fits you, and I believe the fit of a helmet is one of the keys to the protection it gives you. Otherwise, it's best to buy a cycle helmet from a good bike shop, so you can benefit from their expertise and they might help custom fit it for you.

The helmet you buy must be safety certified. At the time of writing, the safety standard for cycle helmets in the UK is the European standard, EN 1078. Make sure that those you are considering meet that standard. They probably do, but ask to make sure. Look for a model that is light and has good ventilation, which means plenty of gaps in its surface to let air in. Ask the shop assistant to explain the ventilation merits of any helmet you like. Modern bike helmets are light and so well designed that after a while you won't notice you're wearing one.

Fit is crucial. The helmet won't protect you to its full potential if it's loose on your head, and if it's too tight it might discourage you from wearing it. The key test is to put the helmet on your head straight and level, meaning the bottom of the helmet is parallel to the floor when you are stood up straight. Do not fasten the helmet straps under your chin yet, just let them dangle. Modern cycle helmets have an internal adjustment mechanism to provide a custom fit. Use the mechanism, which is usually on the back of the helmet, so that the helmet lightly grips your head. Once you feel it's secure, and still leaving the chin strap undone, test the fit by gently moving the helmet forward and backwards, just a little way, on your head. The fit is correct if your scalp moves with the helmet.

The next step is to adjust the straps so that the helmet sits on your head straight and level. Poor strap adjustment will tilt the helmet off level, and that compromises any protection it offers. Cycle-helmet straps are very adjustable, but you might need somebody to help you adjust them until you are familiar with how they work. Your helper can also tell you if the helmet is sitting correctly on your head.

Keep standing up straight with the helmet level on your head, so that the bottom part of it is parallel to the floor. In that position you adjust the helmet straps so that when the strap is secured under your chin, the bottom of the helmet remains parallel to the floor. Adjustment can be quite a fiddly job, and you need to be familiar with how the helmet straps adjust, which is why, if at all possible, you should try to get the helmet correctly fitted in the shop you buy it from. When you fasten the helmet in place with the chin strap, the helmet must fit straight and level, and when the chin strap is secured it shouldn't feel tight, just secure. You shouldn't feel the strap constricting you anywhere at all.

SPARE INNER TUBE, TYRE LEVERS AND PUMP OR OTHER TYPE OF INFLATOR

Urban bikes, hybrids and folding bikes are fitted with heavy-duty tyres. Their e-bike kin are the same. If you are using a road you should fit the heaviest, most puncture-resistant, road-specific tyres you can. Mountain bikes are easier to ride on the road if they have tyres called 'slicks' fitted. Again, buy the most robust and puncture-proof slicks you can. A bike shop will be able to advise.

Puncture-resistant tyres have Kevlar or another protective layer(s) within their construction. You can also double protect tyres from punctures with sealants that coat the inside of the tyre or inner tube, and if the tyre and/or tube is pierced the sealant plugs the hole.

Keeping your tyres inflated to the pressure recommended for the type of tyre you are using helps prevent punctures too, but it requires a bike pump with a pressure gauge, or you can buy a separate pressure gauge. Bike-specific pumps with integral pressure gauges are called track pumps, but they are too big to carry on your bike, so you need a smaller portable pump anyway. You can use the cyclist's rule of thumb, literally, to check tyre pressures. Just squeeze the tyre between your finger and thumb, and a correctly inflated tyre should give a little bit, maybe one quarter of a centimetre, but not much. I'll cover portable bike pumps and other inflators later.

You can reduce the risk of punctures, and it's worth doing so because they are a nuisance. They occasionally happen, however, and you need to be prepared. If you puncture on a commute you have two options. You can carry an aerosol can of sealant that you connect to the tyre valve, and the pressurised can introduces sealant as it inflates the tyre. Theoretically the sealant plugs the puncture and the tyre inflates and stays inflated, but operating these devices is a bit fiddly and the seal doesn't always work – at least that's my albeit limited experience.

The sure-fire solution is to replace the inner tube with a new one (see Chapter 5 for details of how to do this). It's quicker and easier to replace the inner tube with a good one than repair the punctured tube while out on your journey. You can then repair the punctured tube at home, if the hole in it isn't too large or the tube hasn't split. The successfully repaired tube then becomes your new spare. So carry a spare inner tube, as well as tyre levers to remove and replace the tyre.

There are gas canisters you can inflate tyres with, and as I pointed out above some of them will inject a sealant into the inner tube for an on-the-spot repair. However, hand pumps, or bike pumps as they are known, have been around for years. They are tried and tested, easy to use, and they come in all sizes. Small hand pumps, often called mini pumps, are really popular, and I think they work best. They are easy to carry, robust and very efficient.

Most mini pumps come with clips so you can attach them to your bike, but you can carry them in a bag in the pocket of a cycling jacket (I'll cover what to wear later in this chapter). You also need to carry your spare inner tube and tyre levers. Most experienced cyclists carry them in a small under-the-saddle bag. Here's a tip: wrap your spare inner tube in three or four layers of cling film, or maybe a bit of foam rubber. It protects the tube from other items you carry, tyre levers for example, rubbing and possibly damaging it. Check the wrapping every now and again, because it can get rubbed away too.

BIKE BAGS

Cycle commuters often have to carry things to work and back. Things ranging from laptops to books and papers, maybe something to eat if you don't have catering facilities at work or don't want to use them, to all the aforementioned items plus a full change of clothes to wear at work. Even if you don't carry any of these things, I recommend you carry some sort of cycling-specific waterproofs to wear over your normal clothes in wet weather. So you need a bag or bags to carry these things in.

This doesn't matter so much for short commutes, although I'd argue it makes them more comfortable, but it's better to carry any load on your bike rather than on your person. It doesn't matter so much with just a laptop and some papers in a shoulder bag, although in warm weather shoulder bags can make you sweat where they sit on your back. If you are not used to cycling with one, shoulder bags can get in the way when you stop and start. They are fashionable, though, and they are easy to carry when walking.

Rucksacks stay in place better than shoulder bags, but they can also make you a bit sweaty. If you decide on a rucksack to carry your stuff, and that is a relatively cheap option, buy a cycling-specific rucksack because they sit better on your shoulders when you are cycling. Check that the rucksack is waterproof before you buy, and read any reviews you can find about it. You don't want a leaky rucksack.

Bags that fit on your bike come in many forms, shapes and sizes. Saddlebags fit under the bike's saddle and they range from different sizes of under-the-saddle bags, through bags that fit behind the saddle, to the classic cycle-tourist saddle bag that hangs by straps from special bag loops underneath the saddle.

Historically saddlebags were used by British cycle tourists and commuters, while Europeans favoured handlebar-mounted bags. Handlebar bags are used extensively in the UK now, but I recommend you use them as extra carrying capacity rather than primary, because if you have anything heavy in a handlebar bag it can affect the bike's steering and general feel. In fact, any extra weight held high up on a bike can affect its handling, which is why, if you are carrying lots of stuff, pannier bags are the best solution.

Pannier bags, often simply referred to as panniers, fit into metal carriers (pannier racks) which attach to a bike's frame on the seat stays and/or forks. In my opinion, the older style pannier carriers and bags are the best, but they have to be fixed to your bike by bolting them to fixing points that are part of the frame's design.

Touring, expedition and many urban bikes have these integral fixing points, as do some mountain and hybrid bikes. If you are going to carry lots of stuff on your commute or while cycling anywhere, check the bike you buy has these fixing points. They are threaded bolt holes; one set either side of the chain stays up near the saddle, and one on each of the two rear dropouts. Bikes with fixing bolts for pannier carriers also have fixing locations for mudguards on their rear dropouts. Mudguard fixing locations, more commonly called mudguard eyes, are the lower of the two threaded bolt holes on the frame dropouts.

If there aren't any pannier fixing points on your frame and you still want to carry things low down on the bike, there are stuff sacs that fit either side of the forks, plus there is a whole range of bags that attach to bike frames with Velcro straps. You can buy a range of bags and carriers for folding and small-wheeled bikes too.

MULTITOOL

Multitools are like Swiss Army knives for cyclists. They have a body like a penknife, out of which various tools, such as screwdrivers and Allen keys, can be drawn to tackle straightforward adjustments, tighten something up or make simple repairs. It's well worth buying a simple multitool. They usually fit in an under-the-saddle bag, and they are a big help should your bike suffer a mechanical mishap. The chances of this happening are vastly reduced if you maintain your bike well, and we'll look at some basic cycle maintenance and care in Chapter 5, but you never know.

MASKS

During the COVID-19 pandemic, the UK government made it law that people travelling on public transport must wear a mask covering their mouth and nose. This was done as a precautionary measure against the spread of the virus. Wearing a mask when cycling with others around you is something we might all have to do at some point, and cycling-specific masks have been around for quite some time. In fact, many cyclists were wearing masks when cycling around the UK's towns and cities, irrespective of COVID-19, but still with a view to protecting their health.

Prolonged exposure to the sort of pollutants found in the air, which can happen if you cycle regularly in urban areas, can have a bad effect on human health, putting people at risk of developing asthma, bronchitis and emphysema. Exposure to airborne pollutants can worsen the condition of asthma sufferers, who are otherwise able to manage its effects successfully. Having said all that, though, the health benefits of cycling still outweigh the risks and, going forward, if the urban planning changes being promised now come to fruition, then all urban environments should become much cleaner.

Still, wearing a mask while cycling in urban areas with motorised traffic nearby is worth considering. Cycling masks block fumes, road- and building-work dust while reducing pollen inhalation, which is great news for hay-fever and asthma sufferers. Look for those labelled with an N95 or N99 certificate, which are capable of preventing you inhaling 95 and 99 per cent of particles respectively. This includes fine particulate matter (PM 2.5) suspended in the air, which is dangerous because it can stay in your lungs for a long time.

We all have slightly different head and face shapes and sizes, and the mask must fit your face so there are no gaps, but it shouldn't fit so tightly it restricts your breathing. Most manufacturers produce size guides for their masks, and if you buy from a bike shop the staff will help.

LIGHTS

It's crucial not just to be seen, you need to be seen as a cyclist by other road users. They have to be able to immediately identify you as a cyclist, and you must take steps to help them do that by choosing what you wear, and what you put on your bike, so you stand out as a cyclist against everything that's going on in an urban environment. And I don't just mean when it's dark, you have to show up as a cyclist day or night against a backdrop of distractions.

The first words so many cyclists hear after they have been sent sprawling on the ground in a collision with another vehicle or pedestrian are: 'Sorry mate, I didn't see you.' It's not a valid excuse, but it's a fact of life and one of which you must be aware. I'm not trying to alarm you, I'm just telling it as it is so you are always mindful of this fact and take every possible step to be seen on the road.

Wear bright clothing, or a bright yellow or orange safety tabard, or a reflective Sam Browne belt, and a brightly coloured helmet. Flashing lights front and rear are a must for urban cycling. In fact, I recommend you use them whenever and wherever you ride. A little white flashing LED on the front of your bike and a red one at the rear attracts the attention of other road users. The lights prompt them to think, 'What's that?' It prompts them to look harder, and in doing so they identify you as a person who is cycling. So far I'm talking about daylight hours: you need to be even more obvious to stand out as a cyclist in the dark.

UK law says that cyclists riding on the road during the hours of darkness (times are based on sunset and sunrise, so they change) must display a white light at the front of their bike and a red one at the rear. They must also display white reflectors at the front and red at the rear, as well as amber reflectors on the front and back of both pedals.

Most new bikes sold in the UK come with front, rear and pedal reflectors fitted, as well as amber reflectors in their wheels. They are all very useful. Lights and reflectors help you show up from the front and rear, but amber reflectors in wheels help people see you from the side as well. The amber reflectors are useful because, as they are attached to both wheels and pedals, they help identify you as a cyclist on an obvious and maybe even a subliminal level. Amber reflectors indicate that here's something with wheels being propelled by pedals, and in doing so prompt other road users to think, 'It must be a cyclist.' That's how our brain processes things.

The law also stipulates where lights can be fitted (not too low, basically) and the flash rate of flashing LED lights. In any case, common sense tells you not to put your lights too low down on your bike because people won't see them. As for flash rates, the LED bike lights you buy from shops comply. But I think the legal requirement is a minimum for cycling at night. You need to do much more to stay safe.

I've already said you should fit and use a white flashing LED light at the front and a red one to the rear of your bike in daylight hours. At night, I recommend two white lights at the front of your bike, one flashing LED and one constant, and two red lights at the rear. There's a wide variety of front lights, but go for the most powerful you can afford. These often come with separate rechargeable battery packs. As well as helping to make you visible at night, they often have different light-intensity settings, so you can turn up the intensity and see where you are going where there is little or even no street lighting.

Smaller LED lights aren't so expensive, so use one of those in flashing mode on the front of your bike as well as a main constant light. Two red LED lights should be shown to the rear, one on constant and the other switched to flashing mode. You can also buy red or white lights that attach to clothing and to cycling helmets. If you attach extra light to clothing or your helmet, make sure they are white to the front and red to the rear.

Wear some reflective clothing too. Hi-vis safety tabards are a good idea in daylight, but they often have reflective strips to help you be seen at night. Don't buy a bulky hi-vis tabard, like the ones you see outdoor workers wear: you can get cycling-specific tabards, which have good ventilation. Cycling-specific ones are better than tabards runners wear because they are longer, so hang further down your back, helping you stay visible from behind. Gloves with reflective backs are very good at night because they help other road users see your hand signals, which is important.

You can't have too much reflective kit, and in my opinion one of the most useful bits of reflective bike stuff is one of the cheapest to buy and simplest to use: reflective trouser clips. Trouser clips, or bicycle clips as they are also called, are nearly as old as cycling. Originally made from springy metal, they are now mostly plastic and horseshoe shaped, and fit easily but tightly around your ankles over long trousers to prevent the trousers catching the bike's chain and cranks. Anybody commuting in long trousers should buy a pair of bicycle clips. Reflective ones identify you as a cyclist because others see the clips going round and round reflected by their headlights, so they can see you are a cyclist from almost any angle. Velcro-fastened reflective ankle bands are also available.

MUDGUARDS

Mudguards are essential for urban cycling, and if your bike doesn't have mudguards already then get some fitted. There are two types of mudguards: those that attach to threaded fixing points called mudguard eyes on the bike frame, and those that have their own fastenings. The latter are designed to fit bikes, such as race bikes, without mudguard eyes.

Both types usually come with instructions on how to fit them, but bike shops do this sort of thing all the time so ask the shop where you buy them to do it. There might be a small charge, but the shop will fit the mudguards correctly.

Mudguards make cycling in wet conditions much cleaner and more comfortable. Bike tyres flick water up on your clothes and even in your face, making them wet. There is all sorts of dirt mixed in with road spray too. Full mudguards catch almost all of this dirty water.

LOCKS

You will need a bike lock when you cycle to commute or go about your business. Bike thieves abound, it's just a fact of life. There is a bewildering number of locks on the market, and like anything else you get what you pay for. No lock is absolutely thief proof, but professional bike thieves know their business: they know the locks they can break quickly, and the ones they can't. The ones they can't tend to be more expensive. Do a bit of consumer research on the internet before you buy.

Bike locks work by securing the bike to a solid anchoring point, either a custom-made one such as a bike stand, which is increasingly part of our modern urban landscape, or you can lock it to another secure object, such as the metal rails of a sturdy fence. Many businesses cater for cyclists by installing secure bike racks, ether outside or on their premises. Employers are creating secure bike-park areas too.

The next choice is what lock type to buy. The majority of locks fit into either of two categories: fixed or flexible. Fixed locks have a solid bar of metal, often D-shaped, that fits around the bike's frame and an anchoring point, and then is locked in place. With a flexible lock, a thick chain, cable or band, often with some sort of coating, goes around the bike and anchoring point, and is secured by a lock. D-locks often come with carrying brackets that attach to the bike's frame. Some flexible locks have frame attachments, too, or you can carry them in a bag.

INSURANCE

A good lock is a great way to insure your bike against theft, but bikes still get stolen even when they are locked up. It makes sense to insure your bike for its value so you can quickly replace it.

Some home insurance policies include bike theft, but it's better to go to a specialised bicycle insurance company. They can work out a bespoke policy for you that covers accidental damage, emergency bike hire and personal injury, and many companies will fight cases for you if you are knocked off your bike. Search online for 'cycle insurance'.

HANDLEBAR SMARTPHONE MOUNT

These attach to the bike's handlebars or stem and hold your smartphone where you can see it. There are many route-planning apps you can download to a smartphone. A handlebar smartphone mount holds your smartphone securely, and so allows you to follow the route you have either planned or down-loaded on its display and, with some apps, listen to a commentary. More about route-planning apps and route-planning in general is in Chapter 8.

If the traffic is very noisy around you and you can't hear the spoken commentary, use one earbud. Personally I don't like anything in my ears when I'm cycling anywhere because this reduces awareness. In towns and cities, you need to know as much as possible about what is going on around you and, like your eyes, your ears need to be free of any obstructions. One earbud is OK if you are following a route on your smartphone in noisy traffic, but again I'd advise removing it when you are riding on the quieter sections of your journey.

WHAT TO WEAR

This depends on the length of your cycle commute or other journey. If it is short, less than 5 miles, and with few hills, then you can happily cycle in your normal work clothes. You need flat pedals on your bike, trouser clips to protect your trousers, and a chainguard helps there too. You can buy skirt guards to protect skirts or dresses from being caught by the bike's rear wheel.

Footwear

Wear flat boots or shoes to pedal; trainers are OK but some of the bulkier, more cushioned trainers are a bit clumsy for cycling. Even better, get a pair of cycling shoes and clip-in pedals. The problem with cycling in normal shoes is you can only push and not pull on the pedals, so you lose power. Not a problem for most, but if you carry lots of stuff to work and back and ride up a few steep hills, it's worth considering cycling shoes. For longer commutes, 6 miles plus, I definitely recommend them.

The kind of cycling shoes to buy are the ones suited to off-road riding or cycle touring. They have proper walking soles, and the cleats that engage with the clip-in pedals sit in a recess in the sole, so you don't walk on them.

These cycling shoes feel and perform quite like normal shoes, although the prospect of your feet being held on the pedals with the cleats engaged is a bit scary. Don't be afraid. Clip-in pedals are very easy to use but you need to practise with them before you go out into traffic. All you do is place your foot on the pedal and press, and the cleats will click into the retention mechanism on the pedal. There is a retention mechanism on both sides of the pedal, so you don't have to get the right side to clip in. To clip out all you do is twist your foot, heel first, right for your right foot and to the left for the other. Follow the manufacturer's instructions for fitting the cleats to the shoes.

Clothing

If you get any discomfort from sitting on a saddle you can buy padded cycling-specific underwear, but it's easier to fit a gel cover over the saddle for short distances.

In warm weather carry your jacket or other top in a bag, but even in cooler weather a cycling-specific jacket is better. They are cut for cycling, and often have useful pockets for carrying stuff. Get the brightest jacket you can, and one with reflective strips or piping on it.

On the face of it, wet weather presents a cyclist with problems. Cycling in the wet can be uncomfortable, but only if you aren't prepared. The way to prepare is to equip yourself with a light, cycling-specific waterproof jacket and light, cycling-specific overtrousers. The lighter the better, because they roll up easier and fit in small spaces. They need to be waterproof and breathable, which makes them more expensive than non-breathable items but you are investing in your comfort. Just think how much money you are saving by not buying fuel for cars or paying train and bus fares. Non-breathable waterproofs are a pain because you don't have to ride far or make much exertion before you start sweating in them.

For commutes longer than 5 miles you need to start thinking about specialist cycling clothing, and either carrying a change of clothes with you or having them at work. Before I worked from home I would cycle to work and back: this was usually a 10-mile journey but for a while I did a regular 25 miles each way. I tackled both commutes by getting a lift to work on the first day of the week, with my bike and a week's supply of work clothes. I'd ride home that night, then to and from work each day until the last shift, when I rode to work and got a lift home, with my bike and a week's washing.

With specialist cycling clothing you match what you wear to the temperature and whether it's raining or not. Always start with a base layer next to your skin made from a 'wicking' material. Wicking materials absorb body perspiration and pass it to the surface where it evaporates. Cyclists wear them next to the skin because they help to keep it dry, reducing discomfort and the chilling effect of the wind. Wear a thin base layer in summer and a thicker one in winter.

In summer, wear cycling shorts and a short-sleeved top over the base layer. Cycling shorts are padded where you sit on the saddle to provide a layer of cushioning and prevent chaffing. If you are buying shorts in a shop, and I recommend you do for your first pair at least, check the stitching that secures the layer of padding inside the shorts to see that none of it is rough to the feel. If you are trying on shorts remember to bend over to see if they will be comfortable when you are riding.

If you are new to cycling you might think cycling shorts means skin-tight Lycra, but it doesn't. There are normal-looking shorts cut and adapted for cycling, with padding inside to make them comfortable when riding a bike. Even if you have a short commute it's worth buying a pair of these to ride in and carrying your work trousers with you, so you can change when you get there.

If you do buy Lycra the best shorts are bib shorts, which have high backs and loops that go over your shoulders to ensure a good fit. Bib shorts stay in place and don't ride down your back like standard Lycra shorts can. They cover your lower back when you bend into a crouched riding position, which just feels more comfortable.

Cycling tops, called jerseys, have pockets on their backs to carry food or other things. Full-zipped tops are best for summer as you can pull them right down to let the air circulate around you when it's hot. You can buy long-sleeved and short-sleeved jerseys, but if you are only buying one, get short-sleeved and buy some cycling-specific arm and leg warmers. Even in summer it can be chilly riding early in the morning, so you might need something to keep your arms and legs warm.

Arm warmers and leg warmers are extensions to your shorts and top that you can add or remove whenever you wish. They should fit close but be comfortable: buy the kind that have 'grippers' around the top of them. They help hold the arm or leg warmers in place, preventing them moving down your arm or leg as you ride along.

Cycling-specific, thin, sleeveless body warmers with full zips called gilets are very useful too. Slip one over the jersey to combat chilly mornings. They usually fold up small enough to stuff in a jersey pocket when the weather gets warmer. You can use them as a top layer for extra insulation in winter too.

What to wear in winter

Dressing for cycling in winter follows the same principles as summer. Start with a wicking base layer, thicker than you would wear in summer if the temperature is low. Bib tights are long versions of bib shorts made from a thicker textile than Lycra, but with the same fit and wicking properties. Really good bib tights are slightly water-resistant too.

Use a winter cycling jacket on top of the bib tights and base layer. Don't buy one that is too thick because on cold days you can wear your gilet over the winter jacket to increase insulation. This should see you through normal winter conditions in the UK. I don't recommend cycle commuting in sub-zero temperatures. Urban streets are kept mostly clear of ice but patches can still exist, and it's so easy to fall when cycling on ice. If you feel the cold you could add your waterproof as a top layer over the cycling jacket. You'll need it for wet weather anyway. Add or subtract tops as needed to match the temperature.

Feet get cold when cycling in winter, so buy a few pairs of cycling-specific thermal socks. If it's wet you either need spare shoes in your bag, which is true for summer too, or some kind of shoe cover. Neoprene cycling-specific 'overshoes', which is what cyclists call shoe covers, are excellent over cycling shoes. Check they fit over the shoes you wear before buying.

Hands and ears can get cold too. Winter gloves cut for cycling are a must – neoprene ones work best in all weather – and the cycling-specific cut means they are longer than normal gloves so go further up your arms, which stops gaps occurring between the end of your sleeves and the top of the gloves. You can keep your ears and your head warmer with a skullcap that fits under your cycling helmet, but covering your ears reduces your awareness of what's happening around you. Anyway, although they can feel like they are dropping off at the start of a cold ride, most people find their ears warm up quite quickly once they get going.

You'll build up your experience of what works with cycle clothing, but I recommend buying two thermal base layers, some bib tights, a thin winter top, plus a heavier winter cycling top. Add in the gilet you use on chilly spring, summer or autumn days and your waterproof top, and you have a good cycling wardrobe. Your short-sleeved summer tops make good alternative mid-layers. And on mild winter days you can wear your bib shorts and leg warmers.

Gloves

Gloves are a matter of choice in warm weather. Gloves, prefer-ably waterproof, make cycling in wet conditions more comfortable. It's surprising how cold your hands get in the wet, even in summer rain. It's also worth considering the short-fingered gloves that cyclists call track mitts, even if your commute is short. Track mitts help you get a better grip on the handlebars; they also increase your comfort and really come into their own if ever you fall off your bike.

It's natural if you lose your balance to put you hand, palm up, out in front of you. In that situation even a soft fall can result in graz-ing, and a grazed palm is a nuisance. It affects your ability to grip things, which makes cycling difficult, and it just gets in the way of life in general. Track mitts greatly reduce such injuries.

OTHER BITS AND BOBS

Sunscreen

Sunscreen comes in handy when you are riding in direct summer sunlight. Exposed fair skin can quickly burn. This might not be a problem in the morning, but the sun can still be quite intense during a late afternoon or early evening commute. You can buy sunscreens designed specifically for sport. Check the label; they should protect against UVA and UVB light and be sweat resist-ant. If possible, apply sunscreen thirty minutes before exposure, so it soaks into your skin, because that makes it more effective.

Chamois cream

Not every cyclist, even those who ride long distances, needs chamois cream, but it does help some people doing longer commutes who might suffer from what cyclists euphemistically call saddle soreness. Chamois (pronounced 'shammy') cream is a salve that can be applied to the protective pad inside cycling shorts, which used to be made from chamois leather and the name has stuck. Most pads are synthetic now and don't require anything to soften them. If, however, you have a tendency to suffer from saddle soreness or chaffing, and some people do – even Tour de France riders – then chamois cream could the answer.

Lip salve

Wind chill is where the speed of the wind effectively lowers air temperature. It's a bigger factor at low temperatures than high ones, so it's significant in winter. Wind chill can lower the temperature to a point where it can hurt exposed skin, even in the UK. It can cause chapped lips, which is unpleasant. To combat that, smear lip salve on your lips.

AND FINALLY

Remember, all this specialised clothing is for longer commutes, and although some of it can improve your safety and experience on a short commute, you don't need special clothing for the majority of urban bike journeys, 25 per cent of which, research in the UK found, were less than 1 mile.

Chapter 4

....

Are you sitting comfortably?

....

This chapter is about fine-tuning and adjusting your bike so that it is a custom fit for you. We are all built differently. Even people of exactly the same height can have different limb lengths, and limb length as well as height affects how you sit on your bike, and how it should be adjusted to accommodate you.

The extent to which you need to customise your riding position depends on the length of your commute or other journeys you make by bike. If your commute and other journeys are short you don't need the micro-adjustments that somebody riding longer distance does. Just follow the advice in the first part of this chapter to set up your bike so that it fits you.

I recommend that somebody doing a longer commute of 10 miles or more should invest in specialised cycling shoes and clip-in pedals, and they need setting up properly. Ergonomics comes into play a lot more if you ride longer distances, too. The correct saddle height, as well as the saddle's fore and aft position on the bike's seat post, puts you in a position where pedalling efficiency is optimal. It also helps on longer bike rides if your weight is distributed correctly across the bike, so to achieve that you might need to adjust the handlebars.

CUSTOM BIKE SET-UP FOR SHORTER JOURNEYS

Bike set-up addresses the three points of contact with the bike: the pedals, the saddle and the handlebars. We'll look at setting up a bike for short journeys first, considering those three points of contact. The only difference is that bikes regularly ridden over longer distances need a little more precision when addressing how these three point are spaced.

Pedals

You pedal more efficiently and you are more in control of your bike if you pedal with the sole of your foot in contact with the pedal, not your instep or heel. Most people reading this will think what I've just written is obvious, but I don't think it is to everybody. Right from being kids most people when they learn to ride a bike intuitively place the soles of their feet on the pedals, but I think that with some people that intuitive feel for pedalling isn't there. I see people pedalling along with their insteps in contact with the pedals. It's not many, but it's a fact, which is why I'm starting off with the basics.

The way to get your foot contacting the pedal just right is to first visualise the widest part of your foot, which is about 1 centimetre behind the base of your big toe. The widest part of your foot should be directly over the pedal axle. It helps if your saddle is set at the correct height for your leg length, which I'll cover next. Placing your foot on the pedal in the correct position allows all of your leg muscles to push down on the pedal, and it helps your feet pick up the pedals when you set off after stopping, which you'll do frequently when riding in urban areas with lots of road junctions.

Saddle

Right, point of contact number two: the saddle. This needs to be set at the right height above the bike's bottom bracket to allow you to use all of your leg muscles when pedalling. But it shouldn't be set so high that you are stretching your legs at the bottom of each pedal revolution. Also, if the saddle is too high it makes it harder to place one foot on the ground when you stop, and to set off again without wobbling.

To get the saddle at the right height for you, you need to adjust the length of the seat post, which the saddle sits on, that is showing above your bike's frame. Most seat posts are secured in the bike's frame by means of an Allen (or hexagonal) bolt situated behind the top of the seat tube. You will need an Allen key tool to undo the bolt – if you have a multitool there will be one in that. You also need the help of an observer.

Saddle height depends on the length of your legs. At the correct height your leg should be slightly bent when the pedal is at the bottom of each revolution. A sure-fire way of ensuring this is to place your bike against a wall, remove your shoes then get on your bike, supporting yourself on the wall. Now comes the bit you need an observer for. We'll take this in steps.

Step 1. Place the heel of the leg nearest the observer on the pedal, pushing the pedal back and down, which cyclists call back-pedalling, until it's at the low point of the revolution. In that position, your shoeless heel should still be fully in contact with the pedal and the leg should be nearly straight with just a little bit of bend at the knee. You shouldn't feel any pull or strain on the muscles at the back of your thigh. Get your observer to check how your leg looks, and what they see decides whether the saddle must be raised or lowered.

Step 2. To raise or lower the saddle you need to undo the Allen bolt at the top of the seat tube with an Allen key. Once that's done, move the seat post up or down as much as you and your observer think is needed, then retighten the Allen bolt.

Step 3. Repeat steps 1 and 2 until your observer says your lower leg is just as I described in step 1.

Handlebars

To finish off the set-up process we'll look at the handlebars. Do you feel stretched when you are riding? You shouldn't if you bought the correct-size bike in the first place, but how you feel when riding is totally an individual thing. Bear in mind, though, if you are new to cycling it might feel strange at first. If the bike you've got is right for you then you should get used to it.

Give it a few rides but if you still don't feel right with your handlebars and accessing the controls on them, or you feel stretched or cramped, there are things that can be done. You are probably better off letting a bike shop with a good reputation do them for you, though. Just explain that you are new to cycling, and describe how you feel in relation to the handlebars. Shops are getting new customers all the time, so they will listen and try to help.

CUSTOM BIKE SET-UP FOR LONGER JOURNEYS

Pedals and cleats

Feet are the logical place to start when setting up a bike to fit you exactly, but foot set-up is a little more involved when your bike is fitted with clip-in pedals. The position of the cleats that clip into the pedals decides where your foot is held on the pedal. The cleats locate by bolts into threaded holes on the soles of cycling shoes. If the shoes' cleats aren't in the correct place then you won't be able to pedal as efficiently as possible.

Just like riding in shoes without cleats, you need the widest part of your foot to be directly over the pedal axle. If your foot is too far forward you won't be able to transfer the power of your lower leg muscles that flex your ankle joint. If your foot is too far back you lose some of the power of the big muscles that flex your knee and hip joints.

Cleats should be set straight, and unless you know your pedalling is biomechanically perfect you should use a pedal/cleat combination that allows your feet a degree of sideways rotation during each pedal revolution. Again, we'll do this bit in steps, and it's very helpful to have somebody give you feedback so you can get this just right.

Step 1. Put your cycling shoes on then mark where the widest part of each foot is on the outside edge of each shoe upper.

Step 2. Consult the fitting instructions that come with any new cleats, clip-in pedals or new bikes that have clip-in pedals, and make sure you are familiar with them. You should attach the cleats to the shoe so that the centre of each cleat lines up with the mark you made on each shoe upper. Cleats often have lines marking their centre to help you do this.

Step 3. Put your shoes on, engage the cleats with the pedals and turn the cranks until they are parallel to the floor. Ask your observer to look where the mark is on your shoe relative to the pedal axle. It should be directly over it. Dismount and move the cleat until the mark is in the correct position, then fully tighten the cleat fixing bolts.

Saddle

Next you need to set your saddle at the correct height for you. Again, you need the help of somebody to provide feedback to help you get this just right. Here are the steps:

Step 1. Remove your shoes, then using a wall for support place your heels on the pedals. The correct saddle height is when both legs are dead straight at the bottom of each pedal revolution, with the heels still on the pedals.

Step 2. Turn the pedals backwards, which is called back-pedalling, until the pedal on the side your helper is stood reaches the bottom of the pedal revolution and, with your heel on that side still firmly in contact with the pedal, ask your observer to tell you if that leg is straight or not.

Step 3. Loosen the seat-post clamp bolt, and adjust the saddle up or down depending on the feedback your helper gave you, then retighten the seat-post clamp bolt. Repeat this step until your leg is straight at the lowest part of the pedal revolution, with your heel in full contact with the pedal.

Next you need to set the saddle position relative to the pedals, because there is an optimum position for the saddle where sitting on it you can get all the power from your legs into the pedals. You might think, *Why do I need to do that when this book isn't about racing and going fast on a bike, it's about doing every-day journeys?* Of course you are right, that's what the book is about, but losing power means you are putting more effort into pedalling than necessary, which makes cycling harder than it needs to be, and that takes its toll. If riding your bike feels comfortable and relatively easy, and you get to work on time and nicely relaxed rather than tired and wound up, you are more likely to keep doing it. So you may as well try to get this last part of setting up your saddle position right.

When you pedal your thigh is a lever and the saddle is a fulcrum. To make the most of your thigh lever, the saddle should be positioned so that your forward kneecap is over the forward pedal axle when the cranks are parallel to the floor.

Ideally you need a helper to provide feedback to get this right, and you also need a plumb line. I know, not everyone is a keen amateur builder with a plumb line in their DIY toolkit, but you can make one by tying a key or any metal object with a hole in it, such as washers, to a 1-metre length of cotton. Once you've done that, here are the steps for getting the fore and aft position of your saddle set correctly.

Step 1. Put on your cycling shoes. Lean your bike against a wall, get on it and support yourself on the wall. Clip your shoes into the clip-in pedals and back-pedal until the pedal and crank nearest your helper is leading and parallel to the floor.

Step 2. When your forward kneecap is in this position, if you put your hand just behind the kneecap you'll find a small depression on the outside. Place the unweighted end of your makeshift plumb line in the depression and drop the weighted end down until it is on the outside of the forward shoe.

Step 3. Ask your helper to see where the plumb line is in relation to the pedal axle. If it is in front of the pedal axle, move the saddle backwards. If your kneecap is behind the axle, move it forward. You will need to dismount and undo the bolt or bolts that secure your saddle to the seat post to do this. Move the saddle forward or back, then secure the saddle on the seat post.

Step 4. Keep checking until the kneecap and axle line up. When you've finished moving the saddle, check that it is level, either by eye or better still with a spirit level. Once all that's done, tighten the relevant bolts to fix your saddle in position.

If all the above sounds complicated, this is another job a good bike shop will help you with. Many bike shops offer full fitting services, at various prices, but it is worth paying for a good basic fit. This is doubly true if you feel you might enjoy cycling enough to make it a hobby, as well as a means of transport.

Handlebars

The final part of a good custom bike fit for somebody who wants to take on a longer commute, or use a bike for longer journeys, is the handlebars. You want to feel relaxed holding the handlebars, and not too stretched or hunched up. Feeling 'stretched' or 'hunched up' is a bit vague and down to individual perception. Luckily there is a test to check whether this part of your riding position, which we'll call your 'reach', is optimal.

As I said in Chapter 2, road bikes with dropped handlebars are most suited to longer commutes, and this test works best on road bikes. You can do it while riding too. What you need to do is hold the bottom of the handlebars while riding and look at the top of them, the straight bit that is held by the handlebar stem. If the top part of the handlebars obscures the bike's front hub your reach is perfect. If you can see the hub in front of the handlebars, the handlebar stem is too short. If the hub is behind the handlebars, the stem is too long.

If you bought the correct size of bike it will probably pass this riding test. If not, then to ensure your riding position is spot on you need a longer or shorter handlebar stem fitting. You should be able to judge how far the font hub appears in front or behind the top of the handlebars, so you can buy the correct-size handlebar stem. Take the bike to a bike shop and explain what you want; they will be able to supply the correct handlebar stem length and fit it for you.

*   *   *

Some of these adjustments might seem a bit over the top, but they are well worth checking and making adjustments if they need to be made. It will pay back your efforts to do them many times if you are regularly doing 10-mile-plus journeys by bike. Getting everything set up correctly not only helps you ride faster, it will make you more efficient, feel more in control and confident. Plus it will help prevent niggling discomfort or even injury. Riding a bike in the wrong position can put extra strain on knee and hip joints, as well as causing discomfort in the muscles of the lower back and the shoulders.

COMFORT: SADDLES, HANDLEBAR
GRIPS AND OTHER STUFF

Finding the right saddle is crucial to being comfortable on a bike for both men and women. Nowadays new bikes intended for either sex are fitted with gender-specific saddles. If you haven't cycled for some time, however, it's possible that any saddle will feel strange at first.

There's a whole range of new sensory information for a very delicate area of your body to process. Non-cyclists don't sit on anything the way a cyclist sits on a saddle, so it can be a shock at first and you may experience some discomfort. You might even become a little sore until you get used to cycling. This can happen even if you use your bike for short journeys only, but if it does you can buy underwear with padding in the right places to help you, or you could buy a gel saddle cover. Either of those will help you until you get used to cycling. If problems persist, try to find a bike shop where at least one of the staff has some training in saddles and how they fit. They will be able to help and give advice.

If you do longer commutes by bike then you will be far more comfortable and efficient if you wear specialist cycle clothing. If you still have problems then you definitely need the expertise of somebody at a specialist bike shop. As I wrote earlier in the book, bike saddles present particular problems for women, so many bike shops employ female staff who have been trained in saddle fitting, with a whole range of Women Specific Design (WSD) saddles to recommend.

One of the things you feel through your saddle is something cyclists call 'road noise'. It's a nice descriptive term for the constant vibrations from imperfections in whatever surface you are riding over, which are transferred through your bike and up to you. You feel them through two of the three contact points you have with the bike, the saddle and the handlebars.

This can be a problem for some, especially if the streets you regularly ride around are poorly repaired or roughly surfaced. Things are changing, with more smoothly surfaced cycle-specific lanes and cycle-ways planned, but this book is written for today when even some of the cycle lanes the authorities have created are poorly surfaced and not well thought out. There are things you can do to combat this, though.

One of the things gel saddle covers do is absorb or dampen some of the vibrations coming from the road. You can buy gel handle-bar grips too for bikes with flat handlebars. I'll write more about this in Chapter 6: Cycling skills, but you can flex your arms to absorb the bigger bumps and your legs to soften the effects of bumps and knocks transmitted through the pedals. The main thing is to stick with cycling: your body thrives on new challenges and is brilliant at responding and adapting to them. You'll soon get used to the vibrations and hardly notice them.

In a short time you'll only really notice the big bumps in the road, and your body will eventually find ways of coping with those too. I'll talk about how to do this, how to ride over rough surfaces and cope with other possible obstacles you might encounter in our towns and cities, in chapters 6 and 8.

Chapter 5

Caring for your bike

....

In this chapter we'll look at how to keep your bike running in perfect working order, how to spot problems and ensure it is safe to use, how to do some basic maintenance and cycle repair jobs, and how to care for your bike in general.

MAKING SAFETY CHECKS

This is something you should do regularly. Not only does giving your bike a quick once-over check for anything that might let you down and cause inconvenience, or even break and cause a fall, it helps you keep check on what parts are wearing. Regular bike safety checks help save money. Worn parts are weak links, but they also help to wear out the parts with which they integrate.

It's quick and easy to do a safety check every week, and replace any worn parts as soon as possible. You can even do safety checks as you clean your bike, which is another key to caring for your bike and ensuring it runs smoothly. It's worth buying spare brake pads, tyres, inner tubes and brake cables to replace any worn parts. Keep the pads, tyres and brake cables at home, and carry the spare inner tube with you. There are plenty of good bike repair books that show you how to fit them, and how to do other maintenance jobs.

I'll cover the steps you need to follow to clean your bike quickly, easily and effectively, but first you should follow these steps for your regular bike safety check. If you know about bike mechanics, or have a bike repair manual and want to follow the instructions in that, replace any worn parts you find yourself. If you don't, then your local bike shop will carry out the work for you.

Step 1. Check brakes for wear by pulling on the front and rear brakes and pushing your bike forward. If either wheel revolves then the front and/or rear brake pads are worn. There is usually an adjuster on the brake levers or callipers you can use to take up some wear. Once you have used all the capacity of the adjuster, the brake pads need replacing. That's not too difficult a job if you have brakes that act on the bike wheel rims; either follow a bike repair manual's instructions or let your local bike shop do it. Replacing the pads on a bike with disc brakes is a bit tricky, so unless you are confident in what you are doing the bike shop is your best bet for this job.

Step 2. With rim brakes you must also check for uneven brake-pad wear, which is a sign the pads are not contacting the braking surface evenly. This reduces the effectiveness of the brakes, so fit new pads or let your bike shop do it.

Step 3. For bikes with cable brakes check the cable outers, the outer housings of the brake cables, for signs of splitting, and check the actual cables where you can see them for fraying. Frayed cables need changing before you ride again. Worn or split outers reduce the effectiveness of your brakes by allowing dirt in to wear and potentially clog the cables, so get a split outer replaced as soon as you can.

Step 4. For bikes with hydraulic brakes, your owner's manual should have information on the operation of disc brakes. You should check the exposed length of each brake hose for splits or any sign of leaking brake fluid. The evidence might be as little as a single droplet or a smear of fluid on the hose. Leakages require immediate attention by a qualified bike mechanic, who will replace the brake hose with a new one, then replace the hydraulic fluid.

Step 5. Check the whole circumference of each tyre for bulges, cuts or splits. Tyres with bulges, deep cuts, splits or any sort of distortion could blow out. If you spot any of these failures, replace the tyre immediately. Look closely at the tread of both tyres for signs of wear. If the tread is worn, the tyre has lost structural strength and can break down and distort or bulge. A tyre that has been in a skid and developed a flat spot can also be dangerous. Replace the tyre if you see these signs.

Step 6. Inspect the wheel rims next. You are looking for evidence of deep scoring on the rims. Rim brakes gradually wear out rims, especially in winter when there is a lot of grit on the roads that your wheels pick up as you ride along. Be aware of this. Next, look at where the spokes are held in the rims. Cracks in the rim surface around the spokes are a danger sign, too. If you see anything like that, take the bike to a bike shop for a second opinion. Finally, check the spokes. A wheel with a broken spoke doesn't run straight and true. To check the wheels pick up the front of the bike, then the rear, and spin the wheels to see if they are running true. If they aren't then check the spokes. If you find a broken spoke get it replaced. If you don't find one and the wheel isn't running true there is an imbalance of spoke tension, which is a problem brewing. A good bike-shop mechanic should be able to correct the wheel for you.

Step 7. Check the bike's frame for cracks and dents, and check underneath the frame too. Take the wheels out of the frame regularly to check around the dropouts. The dropouts are where the wheels are held in the frame and forks.

CLEANING YOUR BIKE

Bikes are resilient and dependable, provided they are cared for. Although sealed bearings proliferate on bikes today, and they require little maintenance, many parts are still exposed. Water gets in and can corrode these parts, while grit sticks to lubricants and can help wear out moving parts.

Removing old lubricant and grit from your bike's exposed parts to prolong their life is one practical reason for regular bike cleaning. Another is the opportunity cleaning gives you to check your bike and notice any potential faults.

Finally, a clean, well-maintained bike is not only a joy to behold and to ride, it is dependable. And being dependable allows you to cycle without interruptions. Follow this step-by-step guide to clean your bike. It's quick and easy to do.

If you aren't familiar with the names for parts used in this guide, refer back to the annotated bike diagram at the start of the book.

Step 1. Ideally you need a hosepipe and a bucket, but just a bucket will do; access to hot and cold water; some different-sized, stiff-bristled brushes; degreaser; sponges; some form of bike-specific cleaning agent; and bike-specific lubricant.

Step 2. Hang your bike up if possible: this makes it easier to work on and get into all its nooks and crannies. Remove both wheels, then wash any excess dirt off the frame and wheels with water from a hosepipe or warm water in a bucket.

Step 3. Spray the chain and cassette with some degreaser, then with a stiff-bristled brush work the degreaser into the chain links, applying more degreaser if required. Do the same with the teeth on the chainrings, the derailleur gears (see 'Adjusting gears' below) and the cassette sprockets, using plenty of degreaser and brushing hard.

Step 4. Scrub the chain with hot soapy water. Use a specific chain cleaning brush to get the best results. The idea is to remove as much old lubricant from the chain's surface as possible. Scrub the front and rear derailleur gears also.

Step 5. Let the chain dry then lubricate it, making sure to get good coverage. Hold a cloth behind the chain to prevent lubricant spraying all over the place.

Step 6. Using hot soapy water, or a proprietary frame cleaner, clean the rest of the bike. Work the cleaner inside the frame angles, and over the handlebars, brakes and brake levers, the pedals and the insides of the brake callipers, underneath the saddle, under the bottom bracket and around the cable guides. Then scrub the cassette and wheels with hot soapy water as well.

Step 7. Rinse the frame and wheels with water. You can use a hose for this step. Then dry the frame with a soft cloth and check the other components, including tyres, for wear or damage.

Step 8. Polish gives your frame an extra bit of sparkle. Take care not to get polish on the brake pads. Wipe tyre treads and side-walls with a dry cloth and put the wheels back in the frame, taking care to secure them well.

HOW TO REPAIR A PUNCTURE

Step 1. Remove the wheel from the frame, then insert the blunt end of a tyre lever between the tyre and wheel rim. Lever the edge of the tyre over the rim. With the lever still under the tyre secure its other end, which has a hook on it, around a spoke. Insert a second lever and push this around the tyre to lift it off, then remove the inner tube. If the tyre is tight you might need to hook the second tyre lever to a spoke and use a third one to remove the tyre.

Step 2. Lift the tyre completely off the wheel and inspect it inside and out for cuts and anything sticking through it. Remove any object sticking through the tyre by pulling it out from the outside. Thorns frequently do this, although they are less of a problem on urban roads.

Step 3. If you puncture out on the road it's best simply to replace the punctured inner tube for a spare one you should always carry, then repair the punctured one when you return home. That can then be your spare tube on future rides.

Step 4. Inflate the inner tube slightly and, pushing the tyre aside on the rim, press the inner tube valve down through the valve hole in the rim. Work the whole of the tube on to the rim and under the tyre. Return to the valve and push it upwards slightly, then lift the tyre over the inner tube. Work the inner tube back under the tyre so the inner tube rests on the rim. Refit the side of the tyre you removed with the tyre levers so that it sits back on the rim. Then inflate the inner tube.

The next steps show how to repair a punctured inner tube. You can do this out on the road, but I always take a spare new inner tube on any bike ride, and if I have a puncture I fit that one, then repair the punctured one at home. You will need a puncture repair kit – bike shops and many supermarkets sell them.

Step 1. Inflate the inner tube and listen for escaping air to locate the puncture. Mark where it is; most puncture repair kits provide a small crayon to mark puncture holes. Continue working around the whole tube, listening in case there are more holes.

Step 2. Deflate the tube and roughen its surface around the puncture with abrasive. Select a repair patch and spread a thin layer of glue over the roughened area of the tube. Spread it so that the area covered by glue is slightly larger than the repair patch you are going to use.

Step 3. Allow the glue to go tacky, then peel the backing from the patch and firmly press the patch, backside down, on to the glue. Ensure that the patch edges are flat and keep pressure on the patch for about a minute. Most puncture repair outfits come with a stick of French chalk and a means of grating it to a powder. Use it to cover the area of the repair with chalk powder and allow the glue to dry fully. Once the glue is dry the tube is ready to use.

ADJUSTING GEARS

When we talk about gears in cycling, we mean the variable gear ratios with which most bikes are fitted. There are bikes without gears, which are called fixies or single-speed bikes. Gear-shift mechanisms are either located in the bike's rear hub, called hub gears, or they are called derailleur gears.

Because most of their moving parts are inside the hub, hub gears are complicated to put right if they go wrong, so require the attention of a trained bike mechanic. Don't let this stop you buying a bike with hub gears though: they are very reliable and, because all their moving parts are protected from dirt, dust and rain, they are ideal for urban cycling. Many urban bikes are fitted with hub gears.

In this section I will show you how to adjust and maintain derailleur gears, which get their name because to make a gear shift, the mechanisms involved derail the bike's chain from one gear ratio to the other. The front mechanism, generally abbreviated to 'front mech', shifts the chain from one chainring to the next. The rear mechanism (rear mech) shifts the chain from one sprocket (sprockets are the toothed cogs on the rear hub) to the next.

Occasionally the front and rear mechs don't make the gear shifts they should, or don't make them cleanly. There are a few reasons why your bike's front mech isn't making clean shifts, and it may be something a bike shop has to fix. First, though, you can try to reset the front mech yourself. They do go out of whack now and again due to control cables stretching or receiving a knock, and nine times out of ten if you follow these steps you can fix it.

Step 1. Operate the front mech to shift the chain on to the smallest chainring, then use the rear mech to shift the chain to the largest sprocket.

Step 2. Undo the clamp that holds the gear cable in place on the front mech. There are two adjustment screws on the front mech, one marked with the letter L, the other with an H. L is the low-gear adjuster. Screw the L adjuster in or out until the inner side of the front mech cage (the part of the front mech that shifts the chain) is about 2 millimetres from the inner edge of the chain. You have now set the starting point of the front mech's travel.

Step 3. Pull the gear cable through the cable clamp; keep pulling it so it is under tension and with your other hand tighten the cable-clamp bolt.

Step 4. Shift the chain to the largest chainring and the smallest sprocket using the front and rear mechs.

Step 5. Use the high adjuster (usually marked 'H') to bring the outer side of the front mech cage to about 2 millimetres from the outer edge of the chain.

SAFE CYCLING IN THE CITY

Step 6. Check the action by shifting a few times between the chainrings.

So that's your front mech working properly. Let's look at what you can do if you experience problems with the bike's rear mech. Most rear mechs are indexed, which means that for every click of the shifter, either up or down, the rear mech shifts the chain from one sprocket to the next.

To ensure that the rear mech works faultlessly, you need to regularly clean and lubricate the two little wheels, which are called jockey wheels, that the chain runs on when it goes through the rear mech. Degrease and scrub them every time you clean your bike, and introduce a few drops of lubricant to the centre of each jockey wheel.

Occasionally, you may find that the chain does not quite engage with the next sprocket when you make a single shift, or else it skips a sprocket and overshifts. In either case, the rear mech needs adjusting. Follow these steps to do that.

Step 1. Shift the chain on to the biggest chainring and smallest sprocket, then undo the cable-fixing clamp so that the cable hangs free. Where the control cable enters the rear mech there is a knurled barrel. Turn this in or out until it is set at half of its range.

Step 2. Use the high adjuster (usually marked 'H') to line up the rear mech's jockey wheels so they are directly below the smallest sprocket.

Step 3. Once you have lined the jockey wheels with the smallest sprocket, raise the back end of the bike off the ground and rotate the pedals forward. If the chain doesn't rotate smoothly use the H adjuster, turning it in or out until it does.

Step 4. When the chain runs smoothly stop pedalling, then pull the cable downwards through the cable-fixing clamp and re-clamp it.

Step 5. Shift the chain to the smallest chainring and the largest sprocket. Push the rear mech with your fingers towards the spokes. If it moves beyond the largest sprocket, screw in the low adjuster (marked 'L') until the mech stops at the largest sprocket when you push it.

Step 6. Turn the pedals, as you did in step 4, to see if the chain runs smoothly. If it does not, adjust the 'L' in or out.

Step 7. Shift back to the smallest sprocket, then shift upwards through each gear. If the rear mech does not shift all the way on to the next biggest sprocket, screw out the barrel adjuster until it does. If the mech overshifts and skips a sprocket, screw in the barrel adjuster until it stops.

ADJUSTING BRAKES

I'm going to use adjusting calliper rim brakes as the main thrust of the steps to follow in this section, but what applies to calliper rim brakes applies to most other types of brakes you find on bicycles. There are side-pull calliper brakes, cantilever and V-brakes, and centre-pull brakes, all of which work by the pull on a brake lever being transmitted by a control cable to cause brake pads to contact wheel rims and slow the rotation of the rims.

Disc brakes are the other brakes you find on bikes today, which work by the pull on a brake lever being transferred by a control cable or hydraulic fluid to brake pads that contact a disc attached to the wheel's hub. Once in contact with the disc, friction from the brake pads slows the disc's rotation and therefore the speed at which the wheel to which it is attached rotates.

If you have to pull a brake lever too far before the brake bites, then the brakes need adjusting. Brake pads eventually wear out and must be replaced, which for most rim brakes you can do yourself by following these steps. Steps 1 to 2 describe how to adjust for brake-pad wear, and steps 3 to 5 describe how to replace the brake pads on rim brakes when they fully wear out. Disc brake pads are best replaced by a trained bicycle mechanic.

Step 1. How far you have to pull a brake lever before the pads engage with their braking surface is a called 'brake travel'. Excess travel means the pads are wearing. To take up this travel, undo the cable-fixing bolt that secures the brake cable to the brake mechanism.

Step 2. Squeeze the sides of the brake until the pads on both sides are closer to and equidistant from the rim. The brake cable will move through the fixing bolt as you do this. Still squeezing each side of the calliper, tighten the bolt, and when it's tight release the calliper.

Step 3. Brake pads must be replaced if they are worn down towards half their original depth; brake pads often have a line along them marking that halfway depth. Undo the Allen key pad retainer in the brake shoe (the shoe is what holds the pad on the brake mechanism) and push the brake pad out of the shoe. If the pad and shoe are one complete piece, i.e. there is no Allen retainer bolt on the brake shoe, replace the whole pad and shoe unit. Brake pad/brake shoe combos are secured on the brake mechanism by an Allen bolt or a nut: undo this and remove the old pad/shoe combo from the brake mechanism.

Step 4. Insert the new brake pads into their shoes, or place the new pad/shoe combos in position on the brake mechanism and tighten the relevant nuts or bolts that fix them in place. You might have to undo the brake-cable clamp bolt to do this as the new shoes will be much deeper than the old pads you removed. Align the brake pads so they are directly in line with the braking surface, then tighten the cable clamp.

Step 5. Pull the brake on with the brake lever and check to see if both pads simultaneously come into contact with the braking surface on the rim of the wheel. There is usually an adjuster you can use on the brake mechanism to ensure both sides of the brake mechanism are bringing the brake shoes into contact with the rim at the same time. This process is called 'centring' the brakes.

YOUR BICYCLE TROUBLESHOOT LIST

No matter how well you maintain your bike some parts of it will wear, and sometimes the wear only reveals itself when the bike exhibits a problem. The following is a list of possible problems and their causes. You can fix them yourself, and there are plenty of basic and advanced bike mechanic courses available, as well as good bike-maintenance books, or let the mechanics in your local bike shop fix the problem for you.

One little tip about bike shops you should consider: if you want the shop mechanic to fit a new part then buy it from that shop. You might get a bargain part by mail order, but you leave yourself open to the shop making up the difference when they fit it. Plus, and I'll keep mentioning this because it's important, it pays to make friends with a good bike shop. Do that and the staff there will look after you.

PROBLEM	CAUSE
The chain doesn't engage a smaller sprocket or chainring when you activate the relevant gear shift lever.	Either grit has become lodged inside the cable outers or the cable lubrication has dried up.
The chain doesn't engage a larger sprocket or does not run smoothly on it.	The cable has stretched, the rear mech is misaligned or the electronic gear-shift system is malfunctioning.
The chain jumps on the sprockets when pressure is applied to the pedals.	Either the chain has a stiff link, or the chain, sprockets or both are worn, or a chainring may be bent.
When you apply the front brake and push the bike forward, the headset moves forward relative to the head tube.	The headset is loose or worn.
You hear a sudden snapping noise coming from a wheel while riding and/or the wheel no longer runs a true line.	A spoke may have broken.
There is side-to-side play in a wheel hub, or when spinning the wheel the hub makes squeaking or grinding noises.	The hub bearings are worn or, in the case of tight and loose spots, the axle is bent.
When pedalling forward the cassette spins, but there is no drive to the bike.	The cassette body, also known as the free-hub body, is worn.
The brakes are hard to apply, and/ or sluggish to release.	Grit and dirt has got inside the cable outers, or the lubrication on the inner cables has dried.
You have to pull the brake lever a long way before the brakes engage.	The pads are wearing down or the cable has slipped through the clamp bolt.
The two brake pads do not contact the braking surface at the same time.	The brakes are not centred.
The brake pads contact the braking surface without pulling the lever too far, but are ineffective at slowing the bike.	There is grease on the pads, foreign bodies embedded in them, or they are wearing unevenly.

PROTECTING YOUR BIKE
AGAINST BAD CONDITIONS

Cycling in winter can cause your bike excessive wear and even damage, but if you take these simple steps you can protect it. Grit thrown up by wheels gets on to the moving parts of your bike, where it combines with lubricants and sticks there causing excess wear to the parts. Water and salt, which is often used to treat roads when ice is likely to occur, will corrode metal parts. Regular cleaning and replacing old lubricant help prevent damage, but preventing the grit, sand, salt and water reaching the delicate moving parts of your bike in the first place helps even more.

Step 1. Fit mudguards if your bike doesn't already have them. Some race bikes don't have the fixing points on their frames for full mudguards, which is a big drawback if you use this sort of bike for all-year-round urban cycling. But you can buy thin full mudguards with plastic brackets to mount them to a race-bike frame. There are also mudguards that clip to the frame, secured in place with tie wraps, which catch spray coming off the front wheel, and clip to the seat post to catch spray from the rear wheel, but they aren't as effective as full mudguards.

Step 2. Waterproof the bike's main moving parts, particularly those that drive it. You should clean your bike's chain in winter just as often as you do in summer, but where you would apply light lubricant in summer and leave it at that, in winter you add something heavier. So after cleaning your chain as suggested in the 'Cleaning your bike' section, leave the chain alone to let the light lubricant sink into all the links. After two to three minutes apply heavier, bike-specific lubricant all over the chain. The heavier lubricant acts as a sealant, and lubrication all over the chain helps prevent the lighter lubricant washing off quickly.

Step 3. Dribble oil on the moving parts of the front and rear mechs. Use a heavier, wet oil rather than the oil you would normally apply during the summer. Every time you dribble oil like this, first flush out the old oil by dribbling some degreaser on the moving parts and letting it sink in for a few minutes.

Step 4. If your bike is equipped with clip-in pedals you should scrub them really well in winter because grit and road dirt collect on them. Let them dry, then drop a small amount of lubricant on each pedal's cleat-retention system.

CABLE TIES AND CHAIN LINK

We'll end this chapter with something that can help you carry on with your bike journey when things go wrong: the wonderfully adaptable cable ties. Always carry five or six cable ties – they fit neatly inside an under-the-saddle bag and weigh almost nothing.

If a bolt that should secure a component to your bike comes loose and drops out, you can cable-tie the component back in place. The same goes for Velcro straps that hold bags in place: you can replace a broken strap with a cable tie. Cable ties can be used to fix all sorts of bike problems, but only temporarily: you still need to fix the problem properly at your very first opportunity.

Buy a replacement link for your chain in case of chain breakage. At a push, though, a thin cable tie does the job, so long as you don't press too hard on the pedals and you haven't got too far to go.

E-BIKE CARE

There isn't much extra to do when caring for an e-bike. Their motors are either sealed or not serviceable, so if you think there might be a problem with the electric motor or with any of the other parts to do with it, you'll need to take the bike to a good bike shop.

You can extend the bike's battery life by keeping its charge topped up. Never let it completely discharge, and protect the battery from extreme heat by not leaving your bike in direct summer sunlight. Batteries don't like freezing cold either, so keep your bike indoors and try to park it indoors in winter too.

Check electrical contacts every now and again for signs of corrosion, and to see if any are loose. Very rarely, you may have a problem where the motor stops working. If that happens try switching everything off then back on again, like a computer reboot. If the motor comes back to life you can continue the journey, but the fact that it died in the first place means there is a problem and you need the skills of a bike-shop e-bike technician to sort it out.

Chapter 6

....

Cycling skills

....

To kick this chapter off I am going back to basics. It's often said, when somebody revisits something they used to do, 'You'll be fine, it's just like riding a bike,' implying that once you learn to ride a bike you never forget how. And there is an element of truth in that: if you learn to ride a bike when you are young, the balance and muscle memory stays with you for a long time. But the saying assumes everybody learned to ride a bike at an early age, which for a few adults is just not true.

If you are learning to cycle from scratch then get some proper qualified instruction. It's probably a good idea to get a short refresher if you are returning to cycling after a long time as well. The problem is there aren't many schemes in the UK that help adults gain cycling skills. There are some in London funded by Transport for London and there is pressure on the UK government to fund adult training schemes throughout the country. Hopefully that will happen now.

If it does then it will mostly likely be done through Bikeability, which trains schoolchildren to cycle safely. Paul Robison, the CEO of Bikeability Trust, which manages Bikeability's funds delivered to councils around the UK, says he has been 'pushing quite strongly' for the government to incorporate adult cycle training into the Bikeability scheme to help people cycle more, especially following the COVID-19 restrictions on public transport. This hadn't happened at the time of writing but it does seem likely it will soon, so check www.bikeability.org.uk to find a course near you.

If you are reasonably confident about cycling but haven't ridden for a while then practise in an area where there isn't much traffic before you take to cycling on busier roads. Empty car parks and open parkland are good places to do this. Just ride around until you feel confident; do some starts and stops too, and right and left turns. It will all come back to you quickly, but it's worth getting familiar with the bike in a quiet place first, because one of the major assets that help you keep safe when cycling on urban roads is confidence. You get confidence by having all the skills in place, as well as a good understanding of your bike and how it behaves and works.

SETTING OFF

The first skill you need to have down is starting off on your bike from a standing start without wobbling. It's a simple thing, but it's important that you master it before you ride on urban roads with traffic around you. Here's how to do it. I tend to get on my bike with my right foot first, so I'll use setting off with your right foot on the pedal and left on the floor, like I do. Just swap left for right if you get on your bike with your left foot first.

I make sure that the right-hand pedal is in the ten o'clock position as I look at my bike from the left. I get on my bike and place my right foot on the right pedal, then push down on it while I get on the saddle. I then pick up the left pedal with my left foot, and this is where you can wobble a bit. Remember to check what is behind you before you set off, and don't set off cycling until there is a suitable gap in the traffic.

To make sure your bike is stable and goes straight when you set off, take hold of the right side of the handlebars firmly with your right arm, but have your left arm a little more relaxed. It's important not to transfer movements from both sides of your body into the steering, so basically you steer with your right arm for the first pedal revolution before getting going. All this is to keep the bike going straight when you set off. It sounds a bit complicated, but getting on a bike and setting off quickly without wobbling soon becomes second nature.

Setting off is a basic skill but an important one. Having the bike moving off from a standing start, going in the direction you want it to without any wobbling, is a crucial basic safety measure when riding in traffic. The next skill to master is how to control your bike at slow speeds, and to learn how your bike works at slow speeds. Do this before you ride in traffic, and it helps keep you safe when you do.

BIKE CONTROL AT SLOW SPEEDS

A lot of urban cycling involves precise riding at slow speeds, and you have to learn how to balance the bike at slow speeds, because you don't have the bike's momentum to help. The physics of cycling means that as you speed up, the bike's momentum increasingly helps keep it and you balanced. Keep your shoulders relaxed at all times; at slow speeds you use them to make small corrections in your balance.

Think about when you were a kid trying to walk along something narrow. You put your arms out to either side of you, and they moved to help you balance. By doing that you were redistributing your weight to maintain your centre of balance. You didn't have to think about it, you did it intuitively. You can't stick your arms out when they are holding handlebars, so your shoulders come into play and help you keep balance. It's something the body does naturally, which is why you shouldn't tense your shoulders when you ride.

Practise setting off from a standing start until you are confident with it, then practise stopping and putting a foot down, which is another crucial skill. You need to slow to a stop, and just at the moment you come to a full stop, place one foot on the ground. Practise it a few times.

When you are riding slowly it's important that you don't transmit any tightness from your upper body into the handlebars, because it will make you wobble. I know that I'm talking a lot about wobbling, maybe unstable is a better word, but either way it's something you have to avoid doing when riding a bike with other road users around you, and new cyclists are less stable when riding their bikes at slow speeds. Wobbling can put you in the path of another road user, and a wobbling cyclist doesn't inspire confidence in other road users, so they sometimes try to overtake when it's not safe. Relax your arms, and don't lock your elbows so your arms are straight. Straight, rigid arms transfer any bumps from rough road surfaces directly into the handlebars, and that can knock you off line.

Grip the handlebars firmly but don't squeeze them. If you grip tightly the tension from your hands goes into your arms. The term 'flat handlebars' broadly describes all bike handlebars other than the handlebars you get on racing bikes, which are called dropped handlebars. Flat handlebars often have some shape to them, but whether straight or with curves in them you hold flat handlebars at either end, where there are tubular grips to provide a secure and comfortable place to hold on to and steer from. Brakes and gear-shift levers are just in from the grips. Make sure you can reach the controls easily without letting go of the grips. The position of the controls can be adjusted to fit you.

Dropped handlebars are straight at the top where there are held by the bike's handlebar stem, then curve down to another flat section at the bottom. They do this because they were originally designed for racing, and racers hold the lower part of the handlebars to crouch down, which improves their aerodynamics. You have a choice of several places to hold dropped handlebars, but for urban cycling I recommend your place each hand on top of the brake levers on either side of the handlebars.

Cyclists call this position 'riding on the lever hoods'. Modern brake levers are designed to accommodate hands holding them like this. It's the best place to hold dropped handlebars for urban cycling because you can steer the bike very well from there and your hands are close to the brake levers. Modern brake levers for dropped handlebars are designed so you can easily apply the brakes while holding the lever hoods.

With your hands in the same position, you can pull on the brake-lever hoods when you are accelerating. Gear-shift levers on modern bikes with dropped handlebars are integrated with the brake levers, so you can shift gear as well. Holding the lever hoods is also best when you ride out of the saddle to help you get up a steep hill (see Chapter 7).

Whatever kind of bike you ride, learn how your bike handles and feels at slow speed by holding the handlebars and riding straight for a bit to get relaxed, then do some slow left and right turns. Reduce the speed as you gain in confidence, turning slowly left and right. Try some U-turns too – they are a really good way to practise riding as slow speeds. Practise these things to improve your balance on the bike.

CORNERING

In urban areas you'll be cornering at much slower speeds than you do on the open road, but a lot of the same principles apply. The first thing is to control your speed for the corner before you reach it. This isn't such a concern if you are cornering straight after a standing start, which you might do after stopping at a junction, but it is a concern when you have built up a bit of speed.

You should apply the brakes before the corner because a bike tends to track straight under braking, so braking once you are cornering can take you away from the line you want to follow. You end up taking a wider line around the corner than you otherwise would.

Pick a line through the corner; basically that's the path you are going to follow, which ideally should be a curve of sufficient radius to get you round the corner and end up in the position on the road you want to be in. Look into the corner before picking the line you want to follow. Avoid riding over anything slippery on the road, such as spilled diesel on a wet road, or any metalwork on the road surface, such as drain covers. You would be surprised how much oil and diesel end up on the roads. Most of the time it is eventually washed away by rain, but it can build up during a prolonged dry spell, which means that when the first rain falls the roads are very slippery.

Taking corners with a bit more speed requires a different technique. If you pedal around faster corners you risk catching the inside pedal on the floor. So always have the inside pedal uppermost, that's the left pedal for a left bend and the right pedal for a right bend. Keep the pedal in position until the bike is going straight again. This cuts out the risk of the inside pedal contacting the road, which can knock you off your bike.

RIDING ONE-HANDED

Another important thing to practise before riding in traffic is riding with only one hand holding your handlebars. You need to ride one-handed at slow speed when you make hand signals to inform other road users of your intention to change position on the road, such as changing lanes or turning left or right.

It's crucial to make hand signals definite and not let your bike wobble. Other road users are less certain of your intentions if you don't indicate them clearly, and you don't look in control of your bike. It can lead them to make mistakes because they aren't sure what you are doing. Some impatient motorists might try to pass you when it's not safe. It's those experiences that put people off cycling in towns and cities, but you can reduce or even eradicate them if you look in control and make clear hand signals.

To control your bike with one hand, keep your arm holding the handlebars relaxed and elbows bent slightly, ready to absorb any bumps. Practise doing this a bit before moving on to the next skill, which is looking behind you while riding and keeping the bike on a straight course.

It's very important before making any turn or changing lanes, or any manoeuvre requiring a change of position on the road or in a cycle lane, that you know what's behind you. You need to know if anything is coming up from behind to overtake you before you move from the line you are following. If it is, then wait.

You can buy rear-view mirrors for bikes, and they are very useful indeed, but you should always check by turning your head too. This is another skill to practise and master because when your turn your head with both hands on the handlebars, your arms tend to pull unevenly on your handlebars, which can take you off course. Be aware of that.

It's actually safer to temporarily let go of the handlebars with the hand on the same side as you are going to look, which means you are just steering with the opposite arm. You only have to look quickly, and while you do that be mindful of keeping your bike going straight. Raise the leg on the same side as you are looking to the top of the pedal revolution before you do this; if it's at the bottom of the pedal revolution you tend to apply pressure on the pedal and this can take you off course.

Always look behind you before making any manoeuvre, including every time you set off into traffic. It's important to know where other vehicles are around you, and only move when there's enough space in the traffic flow for you to do so. Don't be timid: if there is space then signal what you are about to do and do it. Let others know and understand your intentions, then act on them if it's safe to do so.

Steering straight with one hand while looking behind you is another skill to practise until it is second nature. Only then are you ready to take your place on the roads, cycle lanes or cycleways with others.

*   *   *

Work is being done to create a better urban environment for cyclists, one that will actively encourage more cycling in the future, and the COVID-19 pandemic has accelerated that work, but there is some way to go. Some towns and cities are great for cycling in, others less so, but you can still cycle safely in them if you have the skills.

Not only do these skills keep you safe, they make you confident when riding in traffic, and confidence is important. A careful but confident cyclists is seen and respected by other road users. Get the basics right before you cycle in traffic and you will be much safer, as well as enjoying the experience more.

HAND SIGNALS FOR CYCLISTS

There are two hand signals you need to use all of the time: one indicates your intention to move left or turn left, the other indicates your intention to move right or turn right. Simply put the appropriate arm straight out to the side of you, with fingers together and palm facing front. Sit more upright on your bike so those behind can see you. Practise this signal until it is second nature and you can do it without deviating from your course.

You must look behind you before making any change of road position, and if it is safe to change course perform the relevant hand signal and do it. Be definite, don't dither. Wait for a safe space then make the change; it might be changing position in your lane or switching from one lane to another on a multi-lane street.

If you intend to make a right turn in the UK, you need to move to the right side of the lane or carriageway before you turn. To give other road users plenty of notice of your intentions, have a quick look behind to see if it's clear, make the signal to move to the right and, after checking behind again to make sure you aren't being overtaken, move to the right.

You then need to do this again before actually turning right. Look behind and if it is safe to do so, and there is nothing coming in the other direction, of course, do another right hand signal and turn right. Even if you are at a road junction and waiting for the traffic to clear on either side, when it is clear look behind, then make another quick right hand signal to confirm your intentions.

PEDALLING

There is an element of technique to pedalling. For racing cyclists the act of pedalling is a nuanced affair and something they work on to perfect. Their goal is not simply to push down on the pedals, but to push forward at the top of each pedal stroke and pull back (slightly) at the bottom. They are also able to relax the muscles in their ascending leg at the same time as forcefully contracting muscles in the descending leg.

For general cycling, you don't need to pedal with the same style as a Tour de France racer, but there are elements of good pedalling technique that will help you. The most important is your foot position on the pedal, something I've already mentioned. If you pedal with the soles of your feet in contact with the pedals in such a way that the widest part of your foot is directly above the pedal axle, then good pedalling technique follows from that.

You might find you do this anyway, because for many it's an intuitive action when they learn to pedal on a bicycle. As your ascending leg reaches the top of each pedal revolution you should drop your heel slightly. Doing so means you can push the pedal forward slightly as it passes through the top-dead-centre of each revolution.

Equally, if the toes of your descending leg are pointing down-wards at the bottom of each pedal revolution you push, albeit very slightly, the descending pedal backwards through the bottom-dead-centre of each revolution. These are subtle move-ments, but they save energy and help you accelerate quickly and smoothly, which is a great asset when riding in towns and cities because it helps you keep your place in the flow of traffic.

USING THE BIKE'S GEARS

Hub gears are very similar to the gears you'll be used to if you drive a motor vehicle. You set off in a low gear and operate the controls to shift to higher ones as you accelerate. If you come to a hill or need to stop, you shift to a lower gear so you can pedal up the hill with more ease, or are ready in a low gear to set off when the reason you stopped has gone.

Hub gears are progressive: you go from first to second to third gear and so on, matching the gear ratio to your speed, so you pedal at a comfortable cadence. Around 70 revolutions per minute (rpm), or a bit quicker, on the flat, and a little less when riding up hills is ideal.

I don't expect you to count your pedal revs, but new cyclists often fall into a natural cadence that is much slower by using higher gears than they should. This causes them to labour along, and they can be unstable when moving off from standing starts. It also makes them slow to accelerate.

Does your car protest when you try driving it in too high a gear? It does, and so will your body if you try to pedal in too high a gear all the time. A quick and nimble pedal cadence helps you ride faster, accelerate quickly and cleanly, and places much less strain on your body. Think 'nimble' and 'light' when you are pedalling, and that will quicken your cadence.

The other key thing is to shift to a lower gear in anticipation of needing it. Don't leave it until you already need the low gear. So shift just before you arrive at the bottom of a hill so you are in the lower gear right at the start of the hill. The same goes for corners. If you have to brake to control your speed to take the corner safely you need a lower gear to accelerate once you ride through the corner and go straight again. The most efficient way to do that is to shift to the lower gear just before you enter the corner, then you are in the correct gear for accelerating out of it.

Derailleur gears on a bike with one chainring work sequentially, just like hub gears. You set off in a low gear and shift to higher ones when needed. The complication comes when your bike is equipped with two or even three chainrings. Then you need to think about your gears differently. Look at the cassette, that's the sprockets arranged in size order on your rear hub. A derailleur gear shifts the bike's chain between the sprockets with the rear mech, and between the different-sized chainrings with the front mech. Divide the cassette in your mind: you should use the 75 per cent of the cassette with largest sprockets when the bike's chain is on the smaller chainring, and the smallest sprockets with the bigger chainring when you need higher gears. Think of the chainrings like gearboxes fitted to some off-road vehicles: the large chainring is your high gearbox and the small chainring is the low gearbox.

It's important to use your gears efficiently, and bike chains are at their most efficient when they run in a straight line. That's why you avoid using gear combinations of the biggest chainring with the biggest sprockets, and the smallest chainring with the smallest sprockets. The chain doesn't work efficiently with those combinations, so it will wear out faster and use more of your energy.

Anticipation is especially important on hills. At the start of an ascent, choose which chainring you will use to ride up the hill all the way to the top, if you can see the top. You do that because gear shifts between chainrings while cycling uphill completely break your rhythm. Because there is such a big difference in size between the chainrings, if you shift between them you inevitably have to shift between sprockets to find the ideal gear ratio.

There are a couple more things to consider with derailleur gears, and they are to do with the position of the gear shifters. On most modern road bikes, the gear shifters are part of the brake levers, so it's important that you can operate braking and gear shifting levers easily from the same hand position on the handlebars. This can be a problem if you have small hands. If that's the case, you may need help from a bike-shop mechanic to adjust the angle or position of the brake lever/gear shifter units to better suit your hands.

Finally, avoid shifting to a smaller chainring and sprocket at the same time as it can cause the chain to jump off. If you suddenly have to change to a lower gear, change to a smaller chainring first, then fine-tune your gear selection with the rear mech.

RIDING IN WET CONDITIONS

Wet road surfaces can be slippery because oil and diesel get deposited on them by motor vehicles. This is true to a greater or lesser extent depending on how smooth they are: smooth road surfaces tend to be more slippery.

Wet weather also makes painted road markings and metal drain covers slippery. It's not always possible but if you are cornering on a wet road try to avoid your tyres crossing any painted road markings or drain covers. Just take it slower in general when road surfaces are wet, and really slowly if you can't avoid riding over road markings and drain covers.

Keep in mind how wet conditions affect other road users. Falling rain reduces or distorts a driver's field of vision through their vehicle's windscreens, and it can also affect a driver's distance perception. The same goes for motorcyclists and their visors. You should have flashing lights on your bike to help others see you in any conditions, but this is even more important in wet conditions.

CYCLING ON HAZARDOUS SURFACES

Avoid riding over manhole covers, drain covers and grates, cats-eyes and potholes, but don't suddenly swerve to avoid them or you might drift towards another vehicle or even ride into its path. Look well ahead for these things, and if you have to change course to avoid anything check behind that it is safe to do so. If they are unavoidable, do not tense up or brake suddenly; keep in a straight line but get ready to absorb any shock by flexing your elbow and knee joints so your arms and legs act like the suspension of a car.

If you cannot avoid riding over a pothole, raise yourself off the saddle slightly when you see it and shift your weight back just before the front wheel hits it, and forward just before the rear wheel does. Let your arms and legs flex to absorb the shock coming from the hit. Doing this removes weight from the front then rear wheel, cutting the chances of punctures and even damage to the wheels.

Take care when cornering or descending on cobblestones. It is easy to lose control on a surface such as that, and rough cobblestones can knock you off course. Let your legs and arms absorb the vibrations, and lift yourself out of the saddle slightly when riding downhill over cobbles so your bike can move under you.

If you come to a kerb edge, another obstacle or steps, it's safest to dismount and lift your bike up or down them. You encounter quite a lot of low obstacles, such as dropped-down kerb edges, when cycling in urban areas, so you may not want to dismount all the time. So, as already touched upon in reference to potholes, here's a technique that enables you to keep riding when you are faced with some low obstacles and also protects your bike.

Step 1. Approach the obstacle at a right angle and raise yourself from the saddle. Keep your body loose so your arms, shoulders and legs absorb the shock, reducing the impact on your bike.

Step 2. When the front wheel reaches the obstacle move your body back and pull the handlebars up slightly to reduce the weight above the front wheel, cutting the impact on it.

Step 3. Once the front wheel is over the obstacle, shift your body weight forward so the rear wheel is unweighted.

Practise away from traffic first. This technique is only for cyclists who have practised it and are confident with it. Always dismount and lift the bike if a kerb or other obstacle is too high.

CYCLING IN FOG, ICE AND SNOW

Basically, don't do it. Fog restricts vision for all road users, so it makes it harder to see cyclists. Also, fog can be unhealthy in urban areas, and you can end up breathing in all sorts of bad things. If you must ride, and my advice is don't if it's dense fog, then wear a cycling-specific mask. Icy roads are just plain dangerous: do not even attempt to ride if ice is forecast.

Snow is dangerous to ride on once it has been packed down by other vehicles and after it has frozen, so you shouldn't try to cycle in urban areas if there is going to be lying snow there.

Chapter 7

On the road

Once you are confident with your basic cycling skills you are ready to ride on public roads. Ideally, if you are new to cycling your first rides should be on quiet roads. These can be quiet lanes in the countryside or, if you live in a densely populated area, there are always quiet backstreets to practise road riding.

This is your introduction to riding in places where there will be other road users. Keep the skills from Chapter 6 in mind while I talk about the potential hazards from other road users. The big message is that you must constantly monitor and assess what is happening around you.

At the same time, though, enjoy and appreciate the feel of travelling under your own power. Use your bike to explore more and more of your neighbourhood. After a while, cyclists develop a sort of split screen, one side focusing on potential hazards and what other road users are doing, and the other enjoying the experience. More about that split screen later.

Getting used to cycling on country roads or the backstreets of towns and cities builds confidence, and confidence is very important when you are mixing with traffic in busier places. Being skilful boosts confidence, but so does knowing your rights and the laws that affect cyclists riding on public roads. So before we get further into road riding, let's look at what UK law says about cycling on public roads.

THE LAW AS IT AFFECTS CYCLISTS

You need to know what you can legally do and what you can't do on public roads and cycle-ways. You also need to know the laws concerning cycle safety. I have already covered the laws governing bicycle lights in Chapter 3. The Highway Code contains a mix of law and advice for cyclists, and it is well worth reading through the cyclist's part of it. Knowing the law as it affects cyclists can prevent you from getting into trouble. Knowing the law will also help if somebody is infringing your rights. So the following is a quick summary of what the law says about bicycle legality and cyclists' behaviour.

One thing before I go on, though: there is no such thing as road tax. You hear so many supporters of motor vehicle transport, particularly car drivers, grumbling when cycle lanes are created at the expense of road space for them and saying that cyclists should pay road tax. They are confused, because nobody pays 'road tax'. The tax they are paying for in their vehicle licence is an emission tax, and since no emissions are created during a cycling journey cyclists aren't charged an emission tax. Motorists who go on about taxing cyclists argue that the money they pay to use their vehicles on public roads goes to maintaining roads, but it doesn't. We all pay for maintaining roads and creating new ones through other forms of taxation.

Now I've got that off my chest, to the law. These are the main points you need to know and to abide by when cycling on public roads:

1. A bicycle must have two independent brakes, one acting on the front wheel and another on the rear. The main exception to this is a fixie bike because of its fixed-wheel drivetrain. It's called fixed-wheel because if the back wheel is turning on a fixie bike, so are the pedals: it's like direct drive, a fixie rider

cannot stop pedalling and freewheel. The law says that the fixed-wheel drive counts as a braking system on the rear wheel because your legs can apply pressure to oppose the turning of the cranks. This then slows down the rear wheel, and therefore slows the bike down. It's a bit complicated, but don't worry, all you need to know is that fixie bikes can be used on the road with just a front brake.

2. In general, speed limits on roads apply only to motor vehicles. You cannot get a speeding ticket on a bicycle, but there is an offence of careless cycling, which can be used to prosecute if you have been cycling at a speed judged to be careless. To prove carelessness there would have to be conditions on the road that the speed was inappropriate for, or a consequence, such as an accident that was a result of a cyclist riding too fast. The offence of careless cycling applies to public roads throughout the UK, but there are some local by-laws that say cyclists must obey a stated speed limit. The 20 mph speed limit in London's Richmond Park, for example, applies to cyclists and motorists and there is local signage notifying of that. In areas such as that, you can be prosecuted simply for breaking the local speed limit.

3. Highway Code Rule 68 says you must not cycle while under the influence of drink or drugs, but there is no authorised test to see if a cyclist is above the legal limit of alcohol in the blood. Nobody has the power to breath test a cyclist suspected of being under the influence while cycling. It's left to the reporting authority, i.e. a police officer, to establish that a cyclist was riding while intoxicated. Evidence such as a cyclist weaving all over the road, having slurred speech and/or breath smelling of alcohol would be given to help prove a case.

4. Cyclists can ride side by side. The Highway Code Rule 66 states that cyclists should never ride *more* than two abreast

(side by side), which means riding side by side is legal, and given that two cyclists side by side take up less space than a car, it doesn't affect drivers who overtake. In fact, a group of cyclists riding two abreast significantly reduces the time a motorist spends out of position while overtaking them.

5. There is no obligation for cyclists to use cycle lanes that are part of roads or cycle-ways that are separate from the road. Personally I always use them where they are provided. I do it not just because the lanes are a safer place to ride, but I want to support efforts to change our roads so they better suit cycling. Also, it's not only safer to be out of the way of motor traffic, you are being polite by keeping out of the way of other road users. I accept that a few of these lanes or cycle-ways aren't maintained as they should be, some aren't fit for purpose at the moment, and there are a few isolated examples of cycle lanes that are totally impractical. But that is changing. There are lots of initiatives created by local authorities that will improve infrastructure for cyclists. For now, though, if a cycle lane isn't up to scratch where you ride then you can use the road next to it. It's legal to do so. If the cycle lanes are good, though, in the interests of self-preservation and simply getting along with other road users, I advise using them.

6. All the above laws apply to e-bikes as well as pedal-only bikes, but there is a law that applies just to e-bikes. If the motor fitted to an e-bike is no greater than 250 watts and stops providing assistance when the cyclist's speed exceeds 15.5 mph, then if you are over fourteen you can ride it anywhere you can ride a pedal-only bike. If the e-bike complies with the above conditions, all the laws that apply to pedal-only bikes apply to an e-bike. But if the motor is more powerful than 250 watts and continues assisting at speeds higher than 15.5 mph, the e-bike is classed as a moped, so the rider must be sixteen

years or older to ride it and must wear a motorcycle helmet, and the e-bike must be taxed and insured as a moped.

7. Rule 64 of the Highway Code says, 'You must not cycle on a pavement.' A pavement is defined as a path reserved for pedestrians alongside a road.

8. You must be familiar with all road signs and markings, which is common sense. You must obey them too.

RIDING UPHILL

Hills vary in shape, size and gradient, and the secret to cycling up them is correct gear selection and good technique. The first is obvious, you match the gear ratio to the gradient of the climb, but what do I mean by good technique? The overriding thing when riding up hills, especially when you are commuting to and from work or for other journeys where your bike is replacing motor transport, is to get to the top as easily as possible.

So sitting in the saddle and pedalling in a low gear is the best way up a hill. It's the most efficient and least physically taxing way to do it. But small hills, and short steep sections of a long hill with an otherwise mild gradient, need a little bit more force. Many bikes are equipped with an extremely low gear ratio, but if yours isn't you might meet gradients for which pedalling in a seated position won't get you to the top. You can dismount and walk, which is inconvenient but can be sensible, or you do what cyclists call 'getting out of the saddle'. Pull yourself forward to get your weight over the centre of the bike and push down on the pedals while pulling on the handlebars. Your arms, shoulders and back help your legs power the pedals when you climb out of the saddle. It's hard work though.

I've set out some steps to demonstrate the best technique for tackling hills. Strictly speaking, the steps describe the technique to use when cycling up a long hill with a low to medium gradient, which has a steeper section near the top.

Step 1. Assess the gradient as you approach any hill, select the gear you need to start the climb, and aim to spread your effort equally all the way to the top. The last point isn't easy to master at first, but it becomes easier as you get familiar with the hills you regularly ride up.

Step 2. Start any climb conservatively. Stay in the saddle, sitting upright so your lungs have space to breathe. Find a comfortable pedalling rhythm; remember, a fast pedal cadence is more efficient than slowly forcing the pedals round in a higher gear. Once you have settled into riding up the hill, shift up or down a gear to maintain your quick and nimble cadence as the gradient changes.

Step 3. Hold the outside of your handlebars, but not too tightly. Try to keep your shoulders loose because that helps your breathing. If your bike has dropped handlebars, place your hands on top of the brake levers, on the brake hoods.

Step 4. Concentrate on your pedalling, particularly when the hill gets steeper. If the gradient increases to a point where you can no longer pedal your lowest gear ratio quickly, it's important to get the most power from each slower pedal revolution.

Step 5. If the gradient gets even steeper, and you are already using the bike's lowest gear ratio, start pulling on the handlebars with your arms to help your legs deliver more power to the pedals, but be aware that pulling too hard can affect your steering.

Step 6. For the steepest gradients you might need your upper body to help push down on the pedals, and pull up forcefully with your arms. To do this you get out of the saddle and pull yourself forward to help get the power down into the pedals.

RIDING DOWNHILL

Again, confidence is important when riding downhill, and there is some skill to it. Not as much skill as it takes to ride downhill at race speeds, but here are some things to take on board that will keep you safe. The first thing to realise is your bike is more stable at speed than it is if you ride downhill slowly with your brakes on. Having said that, only ride downhill at a speed with which you are comfortable, ready to adjust it for road hazards and for the traffic conditions around you.

You can control your speed a lot with body position. Crouch low and you will go faster, sit up and you slow down. These changes of position also help keep the bike more stable when descending. Lowering your upper body pushes your bottom towards the back of the saddle, which gives good weight distribution, helping to stabilise your bike. This is very helpful with the next thing you have to consider when descending: applying your brakes.

Raise your upper body before you brake, because it creates a solid, triangular shape on the bike and improves its handling under braking. You can also exert more pull on the brake levers if your arms are a bit straighter, but don't lock them straight, they still need to flex to absorb shocks. Raising your body acts as a sort of air brake too. Take extra care when applying your brakes on a steep descent. Don't grab at the brake levers; slowly squeeze them, applying more pressure as you do. Apply the front brake first, then the rear if you need more braking power.

The steeper the descent the more you can apply the rear brake, but it should still be front before rear. Never use one brake full on. If you need more braking power, divide it between the two brakes, front before rear but more rear the steeper the descent. Always brake in a straight line.

Never descend faster than is safe for the conditions. Use you brakes to control your speed, but raising your upper body, even sticking out your knees, acts as an air brake. If the descent is bumpy or wet you should descend slower than if it is smooth and/or dry. You also need to be extra careful and smooth in applying your brakes when it's wet or the road surface is loose. And brake much earlier than normal when descending on loose or wet surfaces.

UNDERSTANDING OTHER ROAD USERS

Once you have the skills, you understand your bike, know the law and are feeling confident about riding on the road, it's time to think about other road users and understand why they do what they do. This goes for cycling in towns and cities, and in the countryside as well.

Pedestrians sometimes step into the road without looking. Motorists will overtake then have to slow down, or they chance overtaking when there isn't enough room to pass you safely, so they pass you too closely. This happens – it shouldn't but it does. Be aware of it, anticipate it, ride as though it is going to happen and, most galling of all, have patience with it. There is a temptation to overreact when somebody does something stupid that potentially endangers you. Try not to do that, you can make matters worse if you do. Things will get better as more and more motorists switch to cycling.

It's human nature for people to be preoccupied. So as well as focusing on the road you have to watch the pavements. If you see a pedestrian walking to the edge, ask yourself, *Are they looking my way?* If they are not then they might not see you and step out into the road. The best thing to do when pedestrians look like they are about to cross the road is, first, check behind you to see if it is safe to move out, so further away from the kerb. If it isn't safe to move out then slow down until you are sure what the pedestrian is going to do. This doesn't happen often, but it happens. In my experience it happens most often in small villages where there isn't much traffic.

Parked cars are another potential danger. Drivers should check behind them before they open the driver's door to get out, but they often don't. Be aware of this and position yourself on the road so there is at least a car door's width between you and a parked car. If this means the vehicles behind can't get past you, so be it. You have to stay safe and they will have to wait. Be careful but be assertive. Your safety is more important than their time.

Patience is a two-way street. We expect it from drivers so cyclists have to try to be patient with other road users. One of the most maddening things cyclists have to deal with are close-passing motor vehicles. A motorist overtaking a cyclist should leave at least 1.5 metres of space between the nearside of their vehicle and the cyclist. There is lots of publicity about this now, many campaigns, and the police in the UK are trying to enforce this rule, but close passes still happen and you should be prepared for them. That's one of the reasons I've written such a lot about cycling skills and how they need to be practised so you are in control of your bike, because you are confident if you are in control.

Close passes are unnerving, but if you have good control of your bike and are riding in a confident manner you'll cope a lot better if it happens. When you are riding along, do a mental checklist now and again: make sure your shoulders are relaxed, check you aren't gripping the handlebars too tightly, and check that your arms are flexed to absorb shocks. This will help you in the event of a close pass.

Plan your routes well. Go for streets and roads with less traffic, even if that means riding further than you need to. Drivers need better education about the dangers of close passing, that is the number-one cure for it, but you can't educate them yourself. What you can do is cut the number of motor vehicles you encounter with creative route planning. More about that in Chapter 8.

Close passes are one of the many reasons why cyclists shouldn't ride too close to the edge of the road. Roads tend to crumble from the edges, potholes form there and a lot of debris gets washed to the sides. Ride at least half a metre out from the edge. It's your rightful position; a bicycle is a vehicle with as much right to be on the road as any other. Keeping away from the edge also give you a little bit of space to move in the event of a close pass.

Above all, don't overreact to a close pass. It's tempting to rebuke the driver and want to point out what they did. Heaven knows I've done it myself. It's not worth it, though. People get very defensive about their driving, and you only have to listen to the news to realise some tempers are like ticking time bombs. If you want to do something about it you have recourse to the law. It is an offence to pass too closely to a cyclist, and if you think the pass was particularly dangerous, note the vehicle's registration number. Write it down as soon as you can, and it's helpful if you have other evidence. Many cyclists ride with a small video camera attached to their cycling helmet or bike. They are very useful in proving a case of close passing.

You then have two courses of action: report the matter to the police or, in the case of a vehicle being used for business, report it to the business. Close passing needs to be stamped out: it is dangerous, especially if the close pass is on an inexperienced cyclist, and it puts people off cycling who would otherwise do it.

Don't feel guilty about reporting a driver, because you could be saving lives. At the very least you are doing something that may help others get into cycling. That does all of us good. Some drivers are serial close passers, they need to be stopped, so report them and contribute to road safety.

Another thing motorists tend to do, especially on urban roads, is accelerate to overtake a cyclist who was travelling at the same speed as them, then slow down in front of the cyclist. This means the cyclist has to slow down and more drivers are tempted to try to pass. It's frustrating when it happens, but be patient.

I'm convinced that some motorists, when they see a cyclist in front, have a programme running in their heads that says: *A cyclist, they are slower than me in my car [or van or lorry], so I must overtake or they will hold me up.* It's frustrating but, again, show patience.

Here's a personal theory that I think will make this and close passes less common in the future. More and more people are taking up cycling, and in doing so they quickly understand what it's like to be a cyclist on the road. They are suddenly aware of how things look to cyclists, and have an immediate regard for their rights and space. They quickly become better drivers because of the experience. You can even tell if the driver is also a cyclist because they pass other cyclists with more than 1.5 metres of space.

They are also good at the next thing I need to talk about: eye contact. This is a crucial thing for all cyclists to develop. Make eye contact with other road users all of the time, and especially before you manoeuvre. You need to know they've seen you before you do anything. If in doubt, wait for them to move. I'll keep coming back to eye contact.

KEEP WITH THE FLOW

I recommend using cycle lanes if they are there: you don't have to use them by law but, as I have said, I always do. I think that cycle lanes are generally the best option for cyclists. On the road, be very careful of undertaking stationary cars, and don't do it if they are close to the kerb. Somebody could be getting out of the car and hit you with an opening door. Don't undertake goods vehicle either.

Instead, take your place in the traffic flow, and if other vehicles are moving slower than you, and if it's safe to do so, overtake them on their right. Always indicate what you are going to do with the appropriate hand signal, and check behind before you make a move.

Ideally try to ride at a pace that keeps you in the traffic flow. Not so fast that you become a hazard, but at a speed that prevents lots of vehicles overtaking you. It will be hard at first but you will quickly get fitter. Riding an e-bike is a big help with this. They are very good in areas that have lots of other traffic.

Be aware of heavy goods and mass transport vehicles such as vans, lorries and buses. Understand what their drivers can and can't see, and what the vehicles can and can't do. For a start, the driver's view to the front is quite restricted by their height, but their view to the rear is very restricted. Never undertake a lorry, van or bus because you can't guarantee the driver will see you.

Remember this golden rule about every vehicle: if you cannot see their mirrors there is no way their driver can see you. Vans, heavy goods vehicles and buses have large areas behind the driver, either directly behind or alongside the vehicle, that are blind for them.

Large vehicles don't turn in the same way as others. They cannot take corners like motor cars: they have to swing out to get the front of their vehicle through the corner, while the rest of their vehicle cuts the corner either very close to the kerb or even over it. Many cyclists have been caught out by this, and it is the reason why the nearside of any of these vehicles is a no-go area. Never ride up the inside of heavy goods vehicles, vans and buses. Don't do it!

RIDING ON COUNTRY ROADS

This book is called *Safe Cycling in the City*, but as a lifelong cyclist I hope you will use your bike for more than that. Exploring the British countryside by bike is a joy, but cycling on country roads has its own hazards.

Although country lanes may not have much traffic, what traffic there is can be difficult to avoid if the lanes are narrow. There are also some very big agricultural vehicles. Keep your ears and eyes open. If you hear something coming up behind you on a very narrow road with banks on either side, look for a passing place and wait there until the vehicle passes.

Of course, the amount of traffic on a particular road can change dramatically depending on the time of day. Get to know your area, and avoid roads with schools and factories on them, especially at the start and end of their respective workdays.

Watch the pavements in villages. Children and elderly pedestrians often walk out into the road without looking, and others do it too. Actually, you soon learn to tell who is likely to step out in front of you: something about their demeanour or body language tells you. People engrossed by the screens of their mobile phone stepping on to the road without checking if anything is coming is a quite common country hazard. It's a hazard in towns and cities too.

Always slow down around schools. Children get excited and will run across the road without looking to see what's on it. Watch out for children when you pass a line of parked cars as they might be too small to see behind the cars, and could suddenly run across the road.

Animals are particularly unpredictable. Cats will see you and still bolt across the road in front of you. Any dog not on a lead needs watching; even the most placid-looking animal might see something on the other side of the road and decide to catch it or chase it. Game birds, especially pheasants, have a habit of looking like they are going to stay on one side of the road then bolt across in front of you the very second you ride by.

Take extra care riding past livestock. In moorland areas sheep graze freely and cross the road whenever they like. They are a particular danger if you are cycling downhill at speed. If you see sheep near the road, slow down to give yourself time and space to react to what they do.

Finally, let's talk about horses. Always pass them very slowly, whether overtaking or riding towards them. If you are overtaking, and you don't think the rider knows you are there, make your presence known, politely of course. A bicycle bell is very useful, it's just noisy enough to attract attention and not too loud or alarming to startle.

A bell is also useful to signal your presence to walkers on narrow lanes, or if you venture on to a bridleway to do some exploring. Bridleways are off-road paths across country areas that permit cycling. Country lanes can be narrow and bridleways are often much narrower, and two walkers side by side leave little room to pass. A quick ring of a bike bell before you reach the walkers will attract their attention, and they should move aside. It's even nice to give a little warning you will be passing from behind if there is room. A well-maintained bike runs quietly, and it's often a shock for older walkers when they are suddenly passed by one. You might have to ring the bell with a bit more force if you encounter runners in the same situation, as they often run with music playing in their ears.

TOTALLY ATTENTIVE

Be confident, not timid. Your bicycle is a road vehicle and you have as much right to be on the road as any other vehicle. Unfortunately this doesn't mean your rights are always respected, which is why you must ride with care and be totally attentive. It's OK to let your mind wander a little and take in the scenery when you are riding along quiet roads in the countryside, but even then you have to develop a mental split screen, keeping one side for attending to what is going on and the other for your thoughts. With practice, you get quite good at this. A mental split screen is crucial when cycling in urban environments.

Cycling in towns and cities requires all your attention: there is so much happening around you and you have to be aware of as much of it as possible. You develop a primary and secondary focus as your urban mental split screen. Primary focus is the road: its condition, where you want to go, the road signs, what's ahead and what's behind, and what the other road users around you are doing.

You also need to constantly assess the threat level. Is that car too close? Has the driver of the vehicle entering a roundabout from my right seen me? Are the pedestrians on the pavement going to remain there, or do some look like they are about to cross the road in front of me?

You quickly develop good focus and good peripheral vision to help you cope. Still, you need to give yourself time to process what's going on, so adjust your speed to how busy things are. Slow down when a lot is happening so you can take it all in, assessing the threat level all the time. And on the subject of vision, if you have to wear spectacles when you drive you should also wear the same prescription when you cycle. If you don't like cycling in your normal spectacles, or find they slip on your face, you can buy prescription cycling-specific eyewear. Your local optician should be able to sort you out.

I recommend wearing protective eyewear to keep dust and little flying insects away from your eyes anyway. Eyewear also helps prevent your eyes from watering, which can happen in cold weather and certainly happens to hay-fever sufferers. Cycling-specific eyewear is best because it's designed to wrap around your face. Go for eye protection rather than just sunglasses. It's good to have protection in bright sunlight, but your eyes need protecting in dull conditions too. Cycling eyewear is available that has several different lens tints, from sun shielding to plain see-through, which are interchangeable in the same frame. You can also buy eyewear with lenses that adjust their tint level to varying light intensity. Eyewear doesn't just protect your eyes from small particles such as dust: getting hit in the eye by a fly when you are descending hurts, and it can quickly turn into a drama.

Takeaway points

★ Be confident, but defensive. Only act on what you are sure is happening, never second-guess what another road user, be they on foot, two wheels or four or more, will do. A motor vehicle offers its occupants some degree of protection, with a high chance of them not being injured in a slow-speed collision. A cyclist has no such protection. Bear that in mind and stay alert at all times.

★ Mirrors can be mounted on the handlebars to help with rear vision, but you must still turn your head around to check on traffic behind. There are also flip-up mirrors you can attach to your arm, and mirrors on stalks that clip to eyewear. They are all very useful. Anything that enables you to see as much as possible can help keep you safe when cycling in urban areas.

★ I can't labour enough how important eye contact with other road users is. Keep it in mind all of the time, and with everything you do. If you have eye contact with other road users you can be fairly confident they have seen you. When in doubt, let them move first.

★ There are occasions when you must let them move first. For example, if you are waiting at a junction at the give-way line before entering a main road, either to go right or left, and a car from your right is indicating left to turn left into the road you are waiting on, do not move out until that car has begun to turn left. Do not rely on the car's indicators, the driver might not have cancelled them from their last left turn, or might decide at the last minute not to make the turn and carry straight on. Only act on what is happening, not what you anticipate is going to happen.

★ Cover the brakes with two or three fingers on a mountain bike, or place your hands on the brake hoods if you have a dropped handlebar. This way you will not have to move your hand very far if you have to brake quickly.

Chapter 8

Cycling in traffic

Now we are at the crux of this book. All that has gone before should have taken you to the point where you have the skills and confidence to cycle along in our towns and cities. This chapter helps you stay safe while doing it. It will help you cope with all that is going on around you, and it will help give you the confidence to become a safe, careful urban cyclist.

The chapter mainly addresses cycling with other road users around you, so on streets with other traffic, but first let's consider how to plan your urban journeys. They won't be the same route you'd chose to drive. You should avoid busy roads with lots of motor traffic as much as possible, and use cycle-specific roads and lanes whenever you can.

ROUTE PLANNING

Cycle route-planner websites are a big help. Cycling UK's Journey Planner (https://www.cyclinguk.org/journey-planner#) is great. You just put in the postcode of your departure point and the postcode of your destination, then choose either 'balanced' or 'quietest' as your route mode to avoid the busiest streets. The planner then plots a route comprised of quieter roads, many of which are part of the National Cycle Network (NCN), which uses quiet roads and cycle-specific trails. 'Balanced' mode is probably best for commuting, because 'quietest' tends to be a bit longer. There are other websites and GPS devices where you can specify what kind of route you want to take.

There are lots of local authorities creating cycle networks in our towns and cities. Many already exist, and the cycle lanes and cycle-ways are the best to choose for your urban cycling journeys. Many of them are well signposted, and local authorities or various bodies also produce maps and websites with details.

A smartphone is very useful for cycle commuting because you can download route-finding apps to it and mount the smartphone on your handlebars. The Bike Hub Cycle Journey Planner is a good example. It's the route-finding engine of CycleStreets, which allows you to choose between 'fastest', 'quietest' and 'balanced' cycling-route options. As well as a visual display, the app gives turn-by-turn verbal instructions, and unlike more general route-planning apps such as Google Maps, it is cycling-specific. The app favours the quietest roads, backstreets and cycle-ways. It works on iPhone and Android and contains loads of useful information, including the whereabouts of bike shops on your route. Hills are another consideration. Some route planners allow you to specify an 'avoid hills' option when planning a route.

Then there's old-school planning: word of mouth or maps. The sport of cycling's governing body in the UK, British Cycling (BC), has created a 'Commute Smart' series of short videos, which are very useful because they answer common commuter questions and provide handy advice for staying safe on two wheels. One set of advice concerns planning a commuter route, and as well as things I've covered above they suggest 'ask a cyclist', which is a brilliantly simple but great idea.

There are more and more cyclists everywhere, and it's highly likely there are a few experienced cyclists where you work. They will know the quiet roads, the shortcuts and even the more scenic routes. And if your work hasn't got secure bike parking, they will know the best places to lock up your bike so it's safe and secure too.

I love maps. The 1:25,000-scale Ordnance Survey Explorer maps are the best for country journeys, but for urban cycle journey planning the larger-scale city maps, 1:10,000 scale, are better. Sustrans is the body responsible for the National Cycle Network, which is 16,575 miles (26,675 kilometres) of sign-posted cycle routes extending throughout the UK, including 5,273 miles (8,486 kilometres) of traffic-free paths. It produces an amazing range of high-quality maps, which it sells through its online shop (https://shop.sustrans.org.uk/maps-and-guide-books). Sustrans is a really valuable source for both urban and country cyclists.

If the route you have planned is going to be a regular one, such as your daily commute to work, it's best to do a practice run so you can refine it. Wear the same clothes as you will be commuting in, and ride at your commuting speed so you can time yourself. Don't rush, and note whether you got lucky with the traffic lights and any other things that might have affected your journey time. Do the same on the return trip. Now you know how long to allow for the journey.

Try to refine regular routes over time. Replace shared streets with cycle-only rights of way. Adding scenic sections such as parks can increase your enjoyment, but watch out for local by-laws that can affect cycling in parks. The same goes for canal towpaths, which you need to have a permit to cycle on. It's easy to get one, just download permits from this link, and fill in the details yourself: http://www.waterscape.com/things-to-do/cycling/permit. There's a code of conduct on towpaths too, which cyclists must abide by, but the rules are simply good manners and they are also on the Waterscape website. You are supposed to carry the permit with you.

JOINING TRAFFIC

OK, good route planning can help avoid cycling with lots of traffic, but there are few towns and cities in the UK at the moment where you can cycle without being close to some motorised transport. In many places you will encounter lots of motor traffic, but don't let it put you off cycling. There are many things you can do to improve your own safety on the roads.

First, let's consider riding along a straight street, maybe with multiple lanes and with other road users occupying them. Where do you ride? What position do you take up on the road? Your default road position, if you like.

Generally, keep over to the left of the road about half a metre out from the kerb, further out if there are parked cars. If the traffic flow is slow then ride further out still. This keeps you in the traffic flow, which prevents motorists from overtaking and squeezing you to the side of the road. You need to give yourself room to play with if a pedestrian steps into the road without looking, or somebody opens the driver's door of a parked vehicle. You aren't being inconsiderate riding in front of a motorist in this situation. They will still be able to pass you when conditions allow, and all vehicles travelling behind will have a better chance of seeing you.

MANOEUVRING IN TRAFFIC

You will need to make left and right turns in traffic, and sometimes change the lane you are riding in, all of which involve you safely manoeuvring your bike in a way that other road users understand what you are doing. Doing this in traffic requires good observation skills and bike control, as well as clear signalling to other vehicles of your intentions for every manoeuvre. Correct gear selection is also important, as are certain skills that you have already practised, such as getting your feet quickly on to your pedals when setting off, riding slowly without wobbling from side to side, and steering your bike with only one hand on the handlebars.

Be confident and show you are confident. Clear hand signals help do that. Use hand signals before you manoeuvre your bike, including when you are setting off from the side of the pavement and into traffic, when you change lanes and when you turn left or right. Always check behind you before making hand signals to ensure it's safe to make the manoeuvre.

Once you have made sure it's safe, indicating the direction you wish to go or turn with a hand signal makes your intentions clear to traffic behind you. But then it's important to check again to see that those around you have registered what you are doing. Do it quickly, in front and behind you. With practice, you get to tell if another road user hasn't seen you. Eye contact is crucial: try to establish eye contact with those around you.

You will have to make frequent stops and starts when riding in traffic. You need to be able to remove your feet from the pedals quickly so that you can support yourself and your bike while you wait to move on. Don't let that put you off fitting clip-in pedals. The clip-in shoe/pedal systems designed for off-road use, as recommended earlier in the book, detach from and clip into pedals very easily. The shoe soles don't slip when in contact with the road surface either.

If you have to overtake a motor vehicle, do so on the vehicle driver's side. Never undertake between a vehicle and the kerb. One of the biggest causes of accidents is a car passenger opening their doors into a cyclist.

Select a low gear before you stop to help you to accelerate away in a straight line when you get going again. Make sure you can support yourself with one foot on the ground while stationary. When the road ahead is clear, glance over your shoulder, and if it is safe to do so, move off.

THINGS NOT TO DO IN TRAFFIC

Never do what cyclists call track-stands, which are only really possible on fixie bikes anyway. Cyclists doing track-stands balance on their bikes with their feet still on the pedals, but no matter how good somebody is at doing this, it's not a safe practice in traffic. Just the slightest contact from another vehicle is enough to make them lose balance and fall.

Never hold on to other vehicles while waiting.

If traffic is stationary, do not weave in and out of it to avoid stopping; just ride slowly and, if you have to stop, put one or both feet down and wait.

TURNING LEFT

Get into position and follow these steps. If you have to change lanes then follow steps 1 and 2 to make that manoeuvre before turning left.

Step 1. Check behind you to see what the traffic conditions are like. If you have to change lanes before turning left, do so well before the left turn you want to make.

Step 2. Wait until there is enough space for you to move into the lane on your left. When it's safe to change lanes make a left hand signal, and check behind again before you move left.

Step 3. When you are in the furthest left lane, position yourself at least half a metre out from the left kerb, as normal. As you get closer to the left turn, indicate your intentions with a left hand signal. Check behind, and if it's safe to do so move a little further out from the left kerb to prevent any motor vehicle overtaking from behind while you make your left turn.

Step 4. Turn left. Moving out in the road slightly in the road before you turn means you will be in the correct position on the road you turn into, which is half a metre out from the left kerb. Continue on.

TURNING RIGHT

When turning right on a two-way street in the UK you are turning across the flow of oncoming traffic, so it is a little more complicated than turning left. Follow these steps to turn right safely.

Step 1. You start a right turn from the right-hand side of the left carriageway, or the right-hand side of the furthest right lane of a multi-lane street. So you need to make that manoeuvre first.

Step 2. Check behind you. If it is safe to do so, signal right. Keep your hand signal in place and check behind again, then if it is safe to do so move to the right-hand side of the carriageway, or the right-hand side of the furthest right lane. On some multi-lane roads you might have to make this manoeuvre more than once, so do it as described each time.

Step 3. Take up your new position, and as you approach the right turn check behind you again so you know what is happening. Signal right for the turn.

Step 4. Once at the turn you may have to stop before turning right to let oncoming traffic – or traffic coming out of the road you want to turn into – clear.

Step 5. When the traffic is clear, do the right-turn signal again, check behind and if it's safe to do so make your right turn, aiming your bike for the slot you will ride in half a metre out from the kerb on the street you are turning into.

Step 6. You should now be riding in a safe position on the road you have turned into.

SIGNALLING REFRESHER

Making multiple direction signals means that you must be comfortable riding at a wide range of speeds while holding your handlebars with one hand. If you need to reduce speed, brake well before you make your signal. Also, when you look behind to check on traffic, it is easy to veer to the side you are looking. Be conscious of this and steer straight; relaxing the arm that is in contact with the handlebar helps.

While you have to take care as a cyclist, other road users are not your enemy and most will respect your right to be on the road. What other road users need is clear indications from you when you want to change direction, and you must be sure they have seen you. This is why eye contact is a vital aspect of riding safely in traffic.

Try to make eye contact with other road users by looking directly at them. Once you have made eye contact, a glance in the direction you are going can be very effective. Making eye contact with other road users reassures you that your presence has been noted. You must still make any necessary hand signals, but at least now you know that the other person will see them.

POTENTIAL DANGERS

Motor vehicles have blind spots because part of the vehicle's structure blocks vision. Good drivers constantly move their heads to check around these blind spots: it's what they are supposed to do. Unfortunately not all drivers are good drivers, which is a problem for cyclists and why it's important to make eye contact. If you can see a driver's eyes they should be able to see you.

Blind spots are a potential danger to you all the time, but round-abouts, filter lanes and slip roads all make the blind spots bigger because one road or lane joins another at an acute angle. This effectively increases the area of the blind spot around the edges of the windscreen. Be aware of that, and give way to the vehicle unless you see that the driver has seen you and has acknowl-edged your presence: eye contact again. With experience you will be able to tell when drivers have seen you. Until then, or if you are unsure, ride slowly and steadily, and always give way. Remember, always ride defensively.

The majority of road users who do not mind you cycling on public roads are worth working with. Never do anything to lose their respect, or you risk adding to the minority who resent cyclists. When pressed for time, some cyclists are tempted to jump their bikes up on to the pavement, ride through a red traffic light, or they might cycle the wrong way down a one-way street. Although it may seem appealing, and it might be safe, and you might not think you are hurting anyone by doing it, don't do it. Apart from being illegal, anyone who sees you will lose respect for cyclists. Good, competent and courteous cycling helps build a positive and accepting environment on the roads.

Cycling defensively helps you identify potential hazards and avoid them. But if you see another road user who is not concentrating on what they are doing, don't interact with them, just reduce your speed or stop and let them get out of the way. Cycling defensively means treating everything as a potential danger until you can verify it is not. Never take anything for granted.

ROUNDABOUTS

Motorist are used to the higher speeds of motor vehicles, so they may not be looking at traffic on the roundabout. They think that whatever is on there will be gone by the time they are on the roundabout, so they might be looking only at what is about to enter the roundabout. Not all motorist do this but some do. If you are on a roundabout look at where the drivers entering it are looking. If they are not looking at you, take extra care.

Make sure everybody behind you on the roundabout or entering it knows what you are doing. Make clear hand signals and keep watching others that are entering the roundabout. Keep asking yourself, *Where is the driver looking?* If they aren't looking at you, be extra careful and ready to take evasive action.

As with all cycling manoeuvres, be vigilant but decisive on roundabouts. Be clear about your intentions. Stick to the lane markings, and don't cut across them even if there is no other vehicle on the roundabout. Try to establish eye contact and work with other road users. Remember, their vehicle creates blind spots for them too.

CONFIDENCE

Cycling confidently and decisively, but at the same time defensively for your own sake, builds respect with most drivers. It certainly does with most professional drivers in taxis, goods and public service vehicles.

Don't be afraid to take charge of a situation. For example, I move further from the left edge of the road when I come to blind bends or when there is a central island on a two-way road. This prevents a vehicle from behind overtaking me and creating a potentially dangerous situation. But as soon as I am past either of those things, I slow down and indicate to whoever is following that it's safe to pass.

It doesn't hurt to let a motorist go out in front of you at a junction. Be decisive, though: let them know they can move past you. Stuff such as this helps build respect. In general, the standard of driving in the UK isn't that bad. Most people are paying attention, and they are polite, in control and safe. I don't want the information about hazards, and what can go wrong, to put you off cycling in towns and cities. There are bad drivers out there, though, which is why you must always cycle defensively and never stop watching what's happening.

USING YOUR HEAD

You can still make eye contact if you are wearing sunglasses. What you are looking for is whether the other road users have seen you. You can tell that from the direction they are looking. And if they are looking directly at you, it doesn't hurt to nod your head in their direction to confirm your contact with them. You can then make your hand signal to indicate your intentions.

ARTICULATED VEHICLES

As touched upon in the previous chapter, be aware that when cornering, articulated vehicles take a different path to cars, motorcycles and bicycles. Keep well behind, as the trailer and cab take two different paths, the cab moving slightly towards the centre of the lane before turning left, and the trailer's path following at a sharper angle, often nearing and even overlapping the edge of the road. Never overtake on the inside. Never line up at a junction next to a vehicle: stay in the gaps.

Remember that vans and all lorries have a big blind spot to the rear of the vehicle, where the vehicle's solid sides and height block the view from the wing mirrors. Keep your distance at all times. All lorries and some vans don't have rear windows. Remember that if you cannot see the wing mirrors, the drivers cannot see you.

ROAD SURFACE HAZARDS

Road surfaces are not always smooth, far from it in some towns and cities. From time to time you will ride over rough, bumpy roads, and even come across hazards such as potholes, the shallow, and some not-so-shallow, holes in the road. Tarmac roads can break up, especially at the edges. Some concrete roads are laid in sections and although the gaps are supposed to be sealed the sealant gets broken, sometimes leaving a tyre-width gap. And many quieter or minor roads have an uneven surface. Finally, you might come across some old cobbled roads during your bike journeys, and even some new ones, although they tend to be smoother.

Rough tarmac or cobbles require the same technique to ride your bike over them. Once you see the surface ahead, shift into a higher gear than you have been riding in, sit well back, and push a bit harder on the pedals. Don't increase your grip on the handlebars, and think more about guiding the bike rather than steering it. Let your arms flex at the elbow and shoulder joints to absorb the shocks. Wet cobbles are slippery, so ride over them with an extra light touch.

Broken tarmac and rough country roads often have smoother sections you can follow. Look ahead, pick a line and steer your bike around the roughest bits, checking behind you first to see that there are no other road users coming up to overtake you.

CYCLE LANE AND CYCLE-WAY ETIQUETTE

Cycle lanes are lanes for bikes only, or sometimes bikes, buses and taxis, along the outer edges of main roads. They are marked by white lines or different-coloured road surfaces. Cycle-ways are cyclist-only roads, or cycle lanes that are physically separated by something solid from the rest of the road. Some urban streets have been made into cycle-only ways in the UK, and a lot more are planned. Going forward, separation is the best way for active and passive transport to coexist.

Cycle-ways are much safer than sharing the road with motor vehicles. They are also more efficient for cyclists. There is still a threat from motor transport at junctions, though. At junctions you need to watch for motorists turning in front of you. If there is a give-way sign you must give way, but it's often safer to do so anyway.

If the lane shares a road with cars, be sure to watch out for parked cars and, as mentioned above, cars turning right across your path. Some cycle lanes pass the end of drives to private houses or the entrances and exits to car parks or business premises, so take extra care there. You can't depend on everybody being awake and checking before they pull out.

There are some rules, although etiquette is a better word, to follow when cycling on cycle lanes or cycle-ways. The first concerns overtaking. Do it like you would when driving. Stay on the left of the lane, and when you catch a slower cyclist, look behind you, and if it is safe to do so move right and overtake.

Once you are ahead of the slower cyclist move back over to the left of the lane.

Some bike lanes have two lanes, one for each direction separated only by a painted line. Be especially cautious when you overtake, checking ahead as well as behind to see if it is safe to overtake, which means nobody coming towards you and nobody trying to overtake you from behind.

When you are about to overtake it is good manners to let the rider in front know what you are doing. If you have a bell on your bike give it a little ring. Or you can say 'on your right' to warn them, but be careful. You don't know how experienced the cyclist in front is, and suddenly hearing a bell rung behind or, worse still, somebody shouting 'on your right' can make them react by looking over their right shoulder and swerving right. Be gentle with your warnings, and don't overtake too quickly

SPEED

Don't ride fast in urban areas, even on cycle lanes or cycle-only streets. You aren't Mark Cavendish pounding around the streets of Paris on the final stage of the Tour de France. Urban cycling requires cooperation. Make progress, but keep your speed down. Go with the flow of what is happening around you. If you are moving much faster than the other traffic, you aren't giving yourself enough reaction time. Somebody will open a car door in your path or step off the pavement in front of you, and you will not have time to react.

Keep the fast riding for out in the countryside or when you are training to get fitter. I mention getting fitter, because even if you are new to cycling and just decided to do more of your daily journeys by bike, you will get bitten by the bug and want to do more. We'll cover fitness, health and wellbeing in the next chapter.

Takeaway points

★ Make clear signals, but still check on what is happening behind you by turning your head. Every time you make a turn or change your position on the road, you must check before signalling your intentions; then check again before you execute the manoeuvre.

★ Cycling defensively means treating everything as a potential danger until you can verify that it is not. Never take anything for granted.

★ Always try to establish eye contact with other road users.

Chapter 9

....

Cycling to get fit
and stay healthy

....

In this chapter we'll look at why cycling is so good for your health and wellbeing: how it improves your fitness, boosts your immune system, promotes self-sufficiency and enhances self-esteem. It will even make you younger – not in years, I can't do anything about that – but in looks, health and general outlook on life. There's even advice on how to get fitter still.

Human beings are hardwired to exercise. We were hunter-gatherers for most of our history. The development of farming and then technology are comparatively recent human events. Our bodies haven't adapted to a more sedentary life, so we need exercise to stay healthy. That means as much steady-paced exercise as we can conveniently fit in, which is why doing more journeys by bike is so good for you, plus getting a little bit out of breath now and again.

Stay active as much as possible, push yourself a bit harder now and again, and the body responds by getting stronger and fitter, and will remain so for much longer. Exercises that make us breathe hard and involve almost all of our muscles working together, such as swimming, running and cycling, do that, but cycling is the best exercise of all.

Why? Because most of us can ride a bike for much longer than we can swim or run. Plus cycling gives you all the workout you need without exposing your body to the dangers of stress injuries, and it reduces the likelihood of muscle, tendon or ligament strains or even tears, because the bike carries your weight. That reduces wear and tear on your body's chassis while allowing you to push your cardiovascular and muscle engine as hard as you like.

WHY CYCLING IS THE PERFECT FITNESS REGIME

The more you exercise the more fat you lose, so long as you don't overeat. The equation is as simple as that, at least it is for the vast majority of us. Cycling therefore is the most effective way to lose weight for the same reason it's the most effective way to get fit: most of us can ride for much longer than we can do other forms of exercise.

But cycling has one or two other things going for it. First of all, it's possible to include some anaerobic training that really boosts your calorie burn both during and for a while after exercise, but without throwing extra strain on to your body because the bike supports it. You even give your muscles an extra workout, a bit like weightlifting, when you set off and accelerate on a bike, and you do that quite a bit when cycling in towns and cities. Pushing up hills is excellent for conditioning and even building muscles.

Exercise improves blood flow to the skin so your skin stays healthy as you grow older. It also improves muscle tone, but cycling also improves muscle strength, particularly leg and lower back strength. Preserving muscle strength is vital as we grow older. Exercise also optimises collagen production, so can stave off wrinkles. Don't forget sun protection though.

Cycling can give you a younger outlook, especially if you take it up as a hobby as well as a form of transport. Out on the road, cyclists of all ages mix because they share a common bond. If you find you really enjoy cycling, join a cycling club. I've been involved in the sport and pastime of cycling for a long time, and cyclists as a group are some of the nicest people I've ever met.

But cycling doesn't just bridge the age gap in practical ways; it makes us feel younger because it was something most of us did when we were kids. It rekindles the feeling and freedom you felt when you had your first bike, the first taste of speed and of the ability to explore your neighbourhood.

Exercise releases natural chemicals, called endorphins, inside your body, and they make you feel happier. Endorphins have a similar effect to some recreational drugs in that they give you a natural and legal high.

Cycling is time away from problems, space to think, and a chance to experience nature and the primal rush of exercise, and in greener spaces you get more in touch with nature. As your body loosens up and you become aware of what's around you, you begin to revel in the simple joy of moving through town or country under your own power.

Cycling improves your cardiovascular system and helps optimise the balance of good and bad cholesterol floating around in your blood. It helps keep your lungs in good working order, your heart strong and your arteries free of obstructions. Cycling also speeds up food transit, and so reduces your chances of bowel cancer. And it mobilises immune cells so you are better placed to fight infection. Cycling is also a great way to control your weight, and being overweight to varying degrees has been linked to a predisposition to a number of life-threatening illnesses.

It's very rare, other than as a consequence of a fall, that a cyclist tears a muscle or tendon. Stress injuries to bones are almost non-existent too. Both of these things are a constant threat to runners. In fact, in his book *Born to Run*, Christopher McDougall states that statistics show that nearly every serious runner suffers a tear or stress injury every year.

Cyclist can suffer ligament or tendon strains, but almost always these are due to incorrect bike set-up. The only big problem for cyclists comes from the very thing that makes it such a great form of exercise. Your bike carries your bodyweight, which means you don't put your bones under much of a load. That's quite unnatural, because bones need to be loaded to remain healthy and maintain their proper density.

Low bone density can be a problem for people who cycle a lot, but it's a problem with a simple solution. Just add some load-bearing exercises to your training regime, such as light to moderate weight training or easy jogging, and your bones will be healthy. That means you can go on reaping all the other benefits of cycling. Unweighted squats, or better still while carrying a sandbag, and a few press-ups and core-strengthening exercises (search online for how to do them) done every other day will help maintain and even increase bone density. Gardening, DIY and even carrying heavy shopping help maintain bone density too.

IMPROVING YOUR FITNESS

If you do more journeys by bike you are already on your way to improving your fitness. Although serious endurance athletes such as professional cyclists employ many different training modes, it is increasing training volume that has the biggest positive effect on fitness. Most experts in this field agree that an effective overall training regime is 80 per cent steady riding and 20 per cent pushing a bit harder. That's the mix most world-class cyclists, triathletes and runners do.

So doing more cycling, maybe adding a bit extra to your commute home, is the way to improve fitness. It's easy to add a bit of extra cycling every day, and it's a nice, de-stressing way to end the working day by adding a loop through a park or alongside a river, or maybe on a bridleway through a patch of woodland, to your commute home. Just adding any cycling to what you normally do will increase your fitness.

Increasing training volume, not intensity, gives you the biggest fitness return for your cycling effort. So for cyclists that means increasing the amount of time spent riding at a nice conversational pace, or a bit harder. The pace you ride to work and back, in fact. Riding at a conversational pace improves your cardiovascular system, and the development of your cardiovascular system is the main determinant in how fit you are. Improve the cardiovascular system and you get fitter.

The cardiovascular system is your lungs, heart and blood, and it delivers fuel and oxygen to your muscles and organs. This provides energy for muscles and organs to work. The cardiovascular system also carries waste products, notably carbon dioxide (CO_2), away from muscles and organs. It helps maintain your body temperature within its very narrow optimal band. And it transports material and chemicals required for repairing and rebuilding your body.

Increasing the amount of cycling you do improves the way your circulation works by improving the efficiency with which gases are exchanged in the lungs, which means more oxygen is picked up and more CO_2 is taken out per lungful of air. Endurance training in particular increases the size of the heart's chambers, so it pumps a large volume of blood around your body per beat. More intense training increases the strength of cardiac muscle, so the heart is more powerful and has a bigger stoke volume. We'll get on to more intense training in a bit. The main thing for now is that you don't need to do much of it.

Both of these adaptations mean that after a period of physical exercise a trained heart pumps more blood further around the body per beat than an untrained one. Training can also improve the quality of blood. In response to doing more steady-paced cycling your blood volume increases, and then the total amount of oxygen-carrying haemoglobin molecules in your blood increases.

Steady-paced cycling stimulates capillary growth in muscles and organs, including your heart and lungs. Capillaries are the tiny blood vessels in which the blood picks up oxygen in your lungs, and are the final stage of the delivery system to your muscles and organs. Increasing capillary density increases the amount of oxygen that can be absorbed in the blood per lungful of air, and it increases the amount of oxygenated blood and nutrients that can be delivered to muscle tissue, allowing muscles to work harder and repair quicker.

So steady-paced cycling increases the amount of oxygen your lungs can pick up, the volume of oxygenated blood the heart can pump per beat, and the size of the network of blood vessels that deliver oxygenated blood to muscles and organs. Add some hills in, press hard on the pedals from time to time, get out of breath occasionally, and do some load-bearing exercises to improve your muscles and bone density, and you will be a fitter human being. You will also be a healthier one.

EXERCISE AS MEDICINE

'Encouraging more people to engage in cycling is crucial to improving the health of the nation and reducing the prevalence of obesity.' The words of Dame Sally Davies, the Chief Medical Officer for the UK, in 2015.

Cycling as a national health panacea? That's a big claim, but it's true. Take one aspect of health, cardiovascular disease, as an example. Statins are mentioned in the media a lot nowadays. They are drugs, some say wonder drugs. They lower the concentration of low-density lipoprotein (LDL), often called 'bad' cholesterol, in the blood, and bad cholesterol has been linked to narrowing of the arteries and therefore to high blood pressure, strokes and heart attacks.

Statins are so potent that some authorities think that anyone in the general population reaching the age where high blood pressure starts kicking in should automatically start taking them. The thing is, statins are drugs, and as such they have side effects, even if some of them might be autosuggested. Why take a drug when exercise, such as swimming, running and especially cycling, because it is so accessible to so many, has exactly the same effect as statins? It does a great deal of other good too.

Many studies show that exercise lowers bad cholesterol. It also lowers blood pressure and increases the concentration of high-density lipoprotein (HDL), 'good' cholesterol, in the blood, without any changes in diet. But what's more, the harder the exercise, the greater these benefits.

One of the studies was carried out at the Harvard School of Public Health. Researchers compared physical activity levels with biomarkers in 1,239 males in a health study. They discovered that vigorous physical activity decreases a man's risk of heart attack, and they were also able to determine why. The benefits of exercise on boosting good cholesterol levels account for 38 per cent of the decrease, but other important markers included increases in vitamin D, lower levels of 'bad' cholesterol and low levels of haemoglobin A1c.

The biomarker haemoglobin A1c is extra important because it widens the effects of exercise on health. Haemoglobin A1c is important in diabetes, in that high levels of it are a marker for the disease, which is becoming a big problem in the general population.

Regular physical activity can reduce your risk of developing Type 2 diabetes and metabolic syndrome. Metabolic syndrome is a condition in which sufferers have some combination of too much fat around the waist, high blood pressure, low HDL cholesterol, high triglycerides and high blood sugar. It's an unhealthy state that predisposes people to a whole range of illnesses.

In addition the National Cancer Institute in the United States says that regular exercise lowers the risk of developing bowel cancer across the general population by 40 to 50 per cent, and developing breast cancer in women by 30 to 40 per cent. Uterine cancer is reduced in active women. Lung cancer too is lower in active people, although that's probably because they are less likely to smoke.

The other big role exercise plays in fighting cancer is in losing weight. Exercise, combined with sensible eating, rather than strict or fad dieting, will help anyone lose weight. And it certainly guards against obesity, which is another factor in cancer.

Obesity is defined as having a BMI, the ratio of a person's weight to height, of over 30. It's a bit of a blunt instrument for individuals, because very muscular people can have a high BMI and they aren't obese, but it's a workable measure when looking at populations. There is a link between obesity and the risk of developing a number of cancers, including kidney, pancreatic, thyroid, gall-bladder, uterine and oesophageal cancers. Obesity may also be linked to developing other cancers too, but more research is required to be definitive.

Another important health benefit is that people who exercise, even when they don't change eating habits at all and have no significant subcutaneous (just under the skin) fat loss, they still lose intra-abdominal fat. That's the fat that forms deep in the centre of the body and has been directly linked with a higher risk of several diseases, including cardiovascular disease.

We know that exercise creates all the benefits listed so far because of a study on twins and exercise, which factors out a lot of variables that occur in the general population. This research also suggests that exercising helps you look and feel younger.

It was done on identical twins and carried out by the Department of Twin Research and Genetic Epidemiology at King's College

London. Identical twins usually share 100 per cent of their DNA, and in childhood they share a common environment, which removes a lot of the nature and nurture factors that can affect comparative studies.

Researchers found 300 identical twins, asked them to rate their exercise habits on a scale, then took blood samples from each one involved in the study and examined the condition of their white blood cells.

The health of a person's white blood cells has long been accepted as a marker of general wellbeing. In the twins study, it was found that the most active of each of the twins had the most robust white blood cells. And there's more. When the white blood cells were examined more closely, down to the level of individual strands of DNA, the active twin's DNA showed a remarkable difference.

DNA strands have protective caps called telomeres on either end of them. Telomeres are a bit like the plastic wrap on the end of a shoelace and they protect the DNA strand. It's not known why, but every time a DNA strand copies itself the copying mechanism doesn't read all the way to the end of the strand. It slices off a tiny section, but the slice occurs in the telomere, which happens because the telomere doesn't contain any genetic information, so nothing is lost. This works well until the telomere becomes too short to protect the DNA. And when that happens in a cell, the DNA in it dies, so the cell begins to degenerate. In other words, it gets old. So telomere length is a good measure of cell age.

In the twin study, the most active of each pair had the longest telomeres at the end of their DNA strands. Activity in the study was gauged at thirty minutes per day, which isn't a lot of exercise, but according to the study the active group had telomeres as long and robust as sedentary people who were ten years younger. And this regardless of the subject's body mass, gender or smoking, plus several other variables that were taken out. So exercise alone made that difference.

Even in identical twins, who start life with the same length telomeres, the most active of the pair had longer telomeres in later life. So they were biologically younger than their identical twin. They were born at exactly the same time but biologically they weren't the same age.

Understanding metabolic age is quite a new phenomenon. In the past it was thought that physical decline in old age was steady and inevitable. Consequently very few people exercised really intensively past their fifties, so any sort of group that could be studied in large enough numbers to negate the ageing theory was hard to get hold of. It isn't now.

Hundreds and thousands of over fifties and even some over eighties run marathons, race bikes, swim miles or do all three, while others are engaged in other quite extreme physical sports. Study those people and you get a very different picture of ageing.

Dr Hirofumi Tanaka of the University of Texas has studied them, and he says, 'A great deal of the physical effects we once thought were caused by ageing are actually the result of inactivity.'

It's been known for quite some time, albeit from studying people who were older but didn't exercise much, that muscle fibres diminish as people age. This was attributed to a loss of motor units, the nerves that tell the muscles to contract and relax. Put crudely, once the nerve goes the muscle fibre can't fire, so it withers. But then a Canadian study of runners aged sixty-five and over found their leg muscles were full of motor units. More motor units means that a muscle can contract faster and more fully. The Canadian over-sixty-fives had as many motor units as twenty-five-year-olds.

Active older men and women have thicker and stronger bones than similarly aged inactive people, although you have to be careful with cycling here. Bone-density loss can occur in people who do little else but ride bikes, even young people who do little else but ride bikes. Some Tour de France riders have been found to have low bone density. Which is why all cyclists, especially older ones, should add some load-bearing exercise, such as lifting weights or jogging, to their cycling programme. Off-road cycling, because of the jarring effect of rough surfaces, is somewhat beneficial in preserving bone density, certainly more so than if you do all your cycling on roads.

I could go on quoting research that shows how exercise benefits health, prevents disease and pushes back the processes we connect with ageing. In fact, a number of people have written books on the subject, and if you want to find out more I recommend you read *The First 20 Minutes* by Gretchen Reynolds. It's very good at debunking some old exercise dos and don'ts too. But the final thing I want to look at is the effect of exercise on brain health, and particularly on how it might affect dementia.

Exercise has a number of beneficial effects on the brain. The first is something it does throughout the body. It promotes the creation of blood vessels and maintains those that exist already in good health. That means your brain gets all the oxygen and nutrients in needs, and it needs quite a lot to function properly.

At the same time, exercise stimulates the creation of new neurons, the connections within your brain. And failing connections within the brain and poor blood-vessel health are causes of dementia. So, although there are other kinds and causes of dementia, exercise can provide a big insurance policy against vascular dementia.

Exercise also makes you feel better and can give you a more positive outlook, and a more youthful one. Exercise does this by boosting serotonin levels in the brain, and low serotonin is associated with anxiety and depression. Some experiments in treating sufferers of anxiety and depression have shown that exercise works better than drugs.

But the other side of exercise is a social aspect. People who exercise tend to mix with all ages. You see this in cycling clubs or similar groups, where older and younger cyclists enjoy doing the same thing, and that helps broaden both of their horizons. On the other hand, sedentary older people can end up being quite socially isolated.

There's no doubt about it, exercise is powerful medicine. It's one that's likely to be prescribed more and more in the future as new medical students graduate, because they are being taught about its power. The government is on to this too, because faced with having to make budget cuts to balance the books, exercise is very appealing because it's free.

So ride your bike. Do it to save money, the planet and yourself. Never since its invention has the bicycle been hailed as such a saviour as it is now. It's a simple invention with an amazing future. Make the bike part of your life and you will never regret it. I haven't.

Acknowledgements

Thank you to everybody at Little, Brown for making this book what it is. Thanks to all the cyclists, experienced and inexperienced, who helped me work out what is important when considering safe cycling in urban areas. Thank you, too, to all the patient drivers out there, and to the impatient ones; just chill a bit, we'll all get where we want to go. Oh, and buy yourself a bike so you can join us in making the world a better place.

Index

Note: page numbers in **bold** refer to information contained in diagrams.